Andie Dominick

←————————————→

NEEDLES

A MEMOIR OF GROWING UP
WITH DIABETES

←————————————→

A Touchstone Book
Published by Simon & Schuster
New York   London   Sydney   Singapore

TOUCHSTONE
Rockefeller Center
1230 Avenue of the Americas
New York, NY 10020

Manufactured in the United States of America

1 3 5 7 9 10 8 6 4 2

The Library of Congress has cataloged the Scribner edition
as follows:

Dominick, Andie.
Needles/Andie Dominick.
p. cm.
1. Dominick, Andie—Health. 2. Diabetes in children—
Patients—United States—Biography. I. Title.
RJ420.D5D66   1998
362.1'9892462'0092—dc21
[b]   98-21415
CIP

ISBN 0-684-84232-7
0-684-85654-9 (PBK)

"Pamphlets" appeared in altered form in the *Indiana
Review,* vol. 18, no. 2, fall 1995, and in the anthology *The
Healing Circle,* edited by Patricia Foster and Mary Swander.

for my parents

Acknowledgments

For help in preparing this book and for love and support, I send thanks to my parents and my husband and to Elyse Cheney, Gillian Blake, Christina Harcar, Leigh Haber, Virginia Mickunas, Steve Pett, Mary Swander, Joe Geha, Gary Comstock, Fern Kupfer, Andy Gottlieb, Bob and Sue Rezek, Ann Rezek, Holly Johnson, Vicki Bott, Margaret Bancroft, Michele Baughman, Christine Yancey, Daylene Niemeyer, Angie Thorne, Joel Verdon, Dr. H. W. Halling, Dr. T. Weingeist, the Graduate English Department at Iowa State University, and the University of Iowa Hospitals and Clinics.

Contents

Needles

I KNOW ABOUT needles. My sister leaves them everywhere. I fill her syringes with water, transforming them into mini–water guns. I have diabetic Barbie dolls and cook meals for imaginary diabetic friends. I watch my sister give herself shots, and when she throws the syringe into the bathroom garbage can, I grab it. Looking out for my parents, I sit cross-legged on the tiled floor, remove the orange cap from the syringe, and set the point against the skin on my leg. I long to insert the needle into my body. I don't think about how it will feel, but rather how it will look, protruding from my thigh.

It seems like a natural thing, to give shots. My own pancreas works, but I love playing with the needles. I line my stuffed animals across my bed and shoot each of them with a syringe full of water before dinner. I tell them it will only hurt for a second, and they don't have any choice. They need to have insulin in their furry bodies if they want to eat. I understand the rules about when they have to get their shots, and I wrap my fingers around their arms and legs and push the needle deep. Then I feed them.

My older brother and I have water fights with Denise's needles after school. I dig through the bathroom trash can and pull out her syringes. The orange caps stand out against the crumpled, white tissues. I carefully pull the top off, dip the plastic tube into a sink full of water, and pull the plunger back. With three or four tucked in the pocket of my T-shirt, I surprise Brian watching television in the living room. The stream of water spurts from the end of the syringe onto his face and hair. He reaches out his chubby hand and grabs the empty syringe, throws it to the floor. Then he runs to the bathroom and locks the door behind him, pulls more syringes from the garbage can, and fills those up.

When he emerges, I douse him again. We try to see who can get the other one wetter. I always win; I can run faster. And I have been playing with the needles for years, popping the caps off and pushing the plunger down. I squirt him twice in the time it takes him to hit me once. I know how to keep bubbles out of the syringes too. With a tap of my finger, I can get the pockets of air to the top, push them out, and be armed with a loaded syringe. Brian isn't careful enough when he draws the water from the sink, and when he points his weapon at me, only a few drops dribble out at the end. The expression on his round face is always one of disappointment. Like he should be able to get it right by now. He narrows his eyes at the empty syringe in his hand and bites his bottom lip. I give him a moment to fully realize his mistake, and then I pull the spare from my pocket and squirt water into his eye.

SOMETIMES I hide my sister's needles in my backpack and take them to school with me. My friends gather along the fence in the corner of the playground, and I pull them out. The girls carefully take the needles from my hand and remove the caps. They examine the metal points with an expression of wonder and lower their bodies onto the grass. We take turns being the doctor, diagnosing rare diseases, giving our advice, and administering the injections. Pretend shots. We always push the caps back on before pressing the syringe against each other's arms.

We are discreet and never get caught by the teachers. I tell my friends it's just a game anyway. We can't get in trouble because we aren't doing anything wrong. I remind them that my older sister takes her needles everywhere. She keeps them in her purse next to two vials of insulin. Even if a teacher sees us, we won't get detention. But we still keep an eye out for the grown-ups and sit with our backs to the other kids playing on the swings. When the bell rings, I slip the syringes into the deep pocket of my baggy corduroys and head back to class.

All the kids know I have the needles. When older kids ask to see one, I tell them to meet me on the playground at lunch and I'll show them. They surround me as I pull a syringe from my pocket and squat down on the grass. I hold up the plastic tube for them to see, but I don't take the top off. I make them ask. Then when I remove the orange cap, I watch their faces. They narrow their eyes and stare at the tip glistening in the sun. Sometimes they ask if they can take one home. I've even been offered milk money for them. I always say no. I can't trust any-one else with the needle.

Last year I let one of my friends take a syringe home with her. She promised to bring it back the next day, but her mom caught her trying to push it into her younger sister's arm. When the telephone rang in our house that night, I knew I was in trouble. My mother's face grew red as she apologized to the woman on the phone. She told me that I shouldn't be digging in the trash and playing with sharp objects. Not that I shouldn't be taking needles to school or sending them home with other chil-dren, but that syringes aren't toys.

DENISE DOESN'T care if I play with them. Sometimes she just hands them to me, saving me the trouble of digging through the trash. On Saturday nights I watch her get ready to go out. Wear-ing only her underwear, she gazes into the bathroom mirror and runs a thick comb through her long, dark hair. She sprays Jontue cologne all over her body. Then she quickly pops a needle in and out of her thigh. If I'm staring at the syringe in her hand, she'll place the orange cap back on and hold it toward me. I wrap my fingers around it as she turns back to the mirror. She applies mascara and dabs her lips with a piece of toilet paper. I fold my legs under me and balance on the edge of the tub, rolling the thin plastic tube between my fingers. She pulls her tight jeans up over her narrow hips and slips her feet into wooden-heeled shoes. When she climbs into her car and heads out to meet her friends, at a park outside Des Moines, I take the syringe to my room and tuck it deep under my mattress. Under the bedskirt and above the box spring so my mother won't find them. She would be mad if she knew I was collecting them—the needles belong to my sister.

I'm nine years old when the needles finally start belonging to me. Denise has been away at college for two years, and she took the needles with her when she moved. The only syringes left in the house are the ones I've saved under my mattress, and those are falling apart. The needles have broken off and the numbers on the sides have been rubbed away. The kids at school don't ask to see them anymore, and now I play with my other toys.

Denise comes home on the weekends to see me. She teaches me her old high school cheerleading routines, telling me that if I start practicing early, I'll be guaranteed a spot on the squad when I get to Hoover High. The judges will be impressed at how much I already know. Even though I have to wait six years until high school, I love the sound of our voices yelling in unison. Denise tells me the crowds are noisy and I have to be louder than they are. My voice has to carry over the heads of the spectators and touch the Hoover Husky mascot painted above the last bleacher. Denise always reminds me to make my movements quick and precise. This afternoon I just don't have the energy to jump around.

"What's wrong?" she asks.

"I'm tired."

"One more routine," she says, cocking her head to the side and studying my face.

And then I lose my balance when I try to do a handstand. She tells me to do it again, knowing I usually have perfect balance on my own. When I get my legs in the air, she steadies them for me. But my arms buckle and I crash down on my head.

I don't cry.

"Are you okay?" she asks, smoothing my brown hair away from my face.

I just stare at her. Her green eyes squint in the summer sun, and the freckles on her nose are only noticeable because her face is so near mine. The wind blows a long strand of dark hair across her cheek. I am dizzy and she almost doesn't look real.

Denise tries to take me inside the house right way, but I tell her I want to ride my bike for a while first. Alone. For two hours I slowly ride up and down my parents' driveway. In the summer, I ride back and forth, garage to the curb, curb to the garage, all day. Usually I imagine I'm a police officer monitoring the traffic on a highway or I'm on a long road trip to see my grandmother. My brother and I have drawn lines with chalk to separate the driveway into lanes, and we've made parking spaces up next to the garage. My dad cut us signs out of cardboard that say POLICE PARKING ONLY. I write tickets to my friends if they park their bikes in my spot. Most days I pretend I'm chasing bank robbers. But now I think about the way my sister was looking at me when I couldn't do a handstand. A look somewhere between disappointment and concern.

WHEN I FINALLY go inside, my dad asks me to pee in a cup. I know what's going on. Denise has told my father to test my urine for sugar. She stares at my skinny legs as I take the cup from my father's hand and turn my back on her. I blame her for this, and while I'm in the bathroom, I think about mixing water with the urine, diluting it just in case sugar does show up in the test. The water will do something. It occurs to me to just put pure water in the cup, but I know my dad will notice that the fluid is too clear. He's been doing these tests for years. He knows what pee smells like. I hold the cup under the water faucet for several seconds. Weighing my options. Knowing in the back of my mind that eventually the truth will come out anyway. Finally, I pee in the cup and set it on the counter.

The orange cap of a syringe in the trash can catches my eye. It looks out of place now that Denise has been gone so long. She must have given herself a shot in the bathroom today. I sit down on the floor and pull it out. It feels familiar between my finger-tips. I pull off the top and stare at the shiny metal. I want to break it off, but I don't. Instead I set the point against the skin on my bare leg, but I can't get up the courage to push it into my skin. I think about slipping it into my tennis shoe and taking it to my room. But I push the cap firmly back on and throw it into the trash can instead.

I walk past my family in the living room, glancing at them briefly and raising my eyebrows. My mother won't look at me. She is slumped into a chair against the wall. Her broad shoulders are small under her green shirt. She's running her thick fingers through her brown hair as she stares out the window. My sister is perched on the edge of the coffee table and looks up at me. I glare at her, hoping she's sorry now for telling my parents. My dad just winks at me like everything will be okay. Like he doesn't want to conduct the test any more than I wanted to pee in that plastic cup. He steadies his large hand on the side of the chair and eases his tall frame forward. I walk past the three of them and slam my bedroom door behind me.

I hear my dad in the bathroom. I know what he's doing. Mixing five drops of urine with ten drops of water in a test tube. Pulling a tablet from the glass bottle with a rusty pair of tweez-ers and dropping the pill into the solution. Waiting for the color to change. And I know by the soft knock on my door that the color in the test tube is probably orange from too much sugar in my urine. If the test had come back a negative blue, he would have knocked louder.

"Come in," I yell, jumping up and grabbing the miniature blender off my doll's refrigerator, pretending now that I have forgotten about the test. I act like it's any other night and I'm just making dinner for my dolls. I don't even turn around when he opens the door. I put my beanbag clown in his high chair and stir air in the pan on my stove. My father sits on the edge of my bed, rubbing his left temple and staring at me for a long time before he speaks.

"Andie, we're going to have to go to the hospital soon."

I start feeding my clown.

"We don't have to go right away," he says. Then he takes a deep breath. "But we'll probably have to go eventually."

There's fear in his voice and I start to cry. He walks over to me and takes the spoon and plate out of my hand, carries me to my bed, and holds me close to his chest. I press my cheek against the red cotton polo he wears every Saturday. He clutches me tightly to him. I don't know how much time passes, but when I open my eyes, and am finally breathing normally, it is getting dark outside. He starts talking again.

"We can try some other things first," he says. "Maybe cutting sugar out of your diet for a while. We'll see if we can't get the tests back down to negative."

I nod in agreement. I know what he's talking about. We watched a show on television a few weeks ago about two young diabetics who avoided insulin injections by not eating refined sugar. The kids went almost a year without giving themselves shots and had gained weight and seemed to be growing fine.

"It's worth a try. And even if we have to go to the hospital, you know it's going to be okay, Andrea. You know that we'll handle it as it comes."

I nod again, but a lump forms in my throat. I know too much. I realize the difference between playing water games with the needles and owning them. Between longing to put one in my body and having to. And my father knows as he kisses me on the forehead that I'm going to grow up more quickly. Responsibility has entered my life, and I'm going to grow up like my sister did.

"Are you ready for dinner?" he asks.

"I'm not hungry," I reply, exhausted from all the tears.

"Okay, kiddo." He squeezes my hand and leaves without looking back at me. He closes the door softly behind him.

I stare at the wall and remember Denise telling me that doctors used to diagnose diabetes by tasting the patient's urine. If they thought sugar was present, the person had to drink his own urine. Sugar was escaping and the person needed to replace it. Get the sweetness back in their bodies. And diabetics died because there was nothing that could be done for them, especially younger diabetics. Their cases were more severe. Denise told me that the needle was a great thing, a lifesaver. I remember agreeing. I said I would choose the needle over drinking my own pee.

"Hey there," Denise says, tapping on the door with her knuckle while she opens it.

I ignore her.

"You gonna lie in here all night?" she asks. "Why don't we take a walk, just you and me?"

I turn my head to the wall and stare at a single rose on my wallpaper.

"Are you mad at me?" she asks.

"Why'd you tell them?" I reply, my voice cracking. "You didn't have to go telling Dad before you asked me. You didn't have to tattle just because I couldn't do a handstand."

She slowly lets all of the air out of her lungs. "Maybe you're right. It's just that you'll feel a lot better after we get you to see a doctor. They can make you better."

"I don't feel bad now," I reply.

I won't turn my head, but I know she's looking around my room, trying to think of something to say.

"Go back to school," I tell her.

"Come on, Andie," she says. The springs of my mattress squeak as she lowers herself onto the bed. I inch closer to the wall.

"Leave me alone."

Denise has given me her disease. It's been hers for almost twenty years, and now it's mine. My mother has told me the stories of Denise's childhood. She was only two years old when she got diabetes. My parents say the doctors and nurses didn't know anything in 1962. It was like Denise was the first diabetic child the hospital had ever treated. My mother describes it as one disaster after another—trying to get my sister to sit still for the painful injections every day, having trouble getting her blood sugars regulated. Denise was in the hospital for twenty-one days.

My parents left there feeling like they knew nothing. They learned about diabetes on their own, checking out books from the library and contacting pediatric doctors around the country with questions. My parents were scared, and they thought Denise was going to die. Eventually they learned how to control the disease, but they didn't know how to control my screaming sister at home. She cried every day when it was time for her shots. Before my father left for the office in the morning, he set my sister on the kitchen table and held on to her while my mom stuck the needle into Denise's skinny leg. Then they gave her another shot before dinner. My mother says they didn't have any choice. Those first needles were like nails.

They used a large glass hypodermic syringe. My mother boiled it in water once a week for five minutes and stored it in a jar of alcohol. Twice a day she pulled it from the jar and pumped it dry before filling it with insulin. She used that same syringe for years. The needle grew dull, and it was hard to get it into my sister's leg, but no one would sell disposable needles to the public. It got harder and harder to get the point through Denise's skin, and my mother finally begged a supply company to sell her some disposable needles. The representative on the phone felt bad, said he couldn't imagine a child that young in so much pain. He finally sold my mom the needles.

Those were sharper, but they were still thick. And Denise still screamed when my father set her on the table. When she figured out that screaming wasn't going to put an end to the injections, she started running from my parents. Instead of chasing after her, they would go ahead with dinner and wait for Denise to come out. She knew she couldn't eat until the needle was pushed into her flesh. Finally, she would appear in the doorway of the kitchen. My dad pushed their plates back and set my sister on the round oak table. My mom grabbed the syringe before Denise could change her mind.

My parents kept notes on everything back then. My mother wrote down what Denise ate at every meal, what color the solution in the test tube was, when Denise had insulin reactions, how much insulin they gave her. The insulin wasn't as concentrated as it is now, so the big syringe was full of the fluid when they put the needle into my sister's leg. My mom taped charts to the refrigerator and then took them to the doctor. For years she wrote down everything. She still has all the old charts buried underneath magazine articles and papers in the basement.

Sometimes my sister hid the syringe. She would climb up onto the kitchen countertop and pull it out of the jar, carry it off to her room. My father knew where to find it. Running his hands carefully over the carpet under her bed, he'd pull the syringe out from between books and stuffed animals. Back to the jar of alcohol it went. This went on until she was six. Then she started giving her own shots. And as she grew up, the needles became thinner and sharper. Now the packages read "microfine" and "designed for comfort." These are the thin needles I used to play with. The ones my sister owned.

MY SISTER and I look alike. My mom digs out old pictures and shows me the resemblance. We both have green, squinty eyes. Our noses are the same shape. My mom says that when I was little, I did things that reminded her of my sister all the time. My teachers call me Denise by accident. They look down at their attendance sheets, see the last name, and call me Denise. They say something about how quickly time passes.

This bedroom used to be Denise's. She picked out this wallpaper with the pink roses on her sixth birthday—years before I was born. My mother has told me the story of how this room became mine. When my mom got pregnant with me, Denise started rearranging the furniture in this bedroom, telling them that she was going to share her room with her little sister. My sister said she knew it was going to be a girl. God would not make her live with another brother like Brian. When my parents laughed and told her I should have my own room, she moved upstairs next door to Brian, saying she agreed the baby should probably be in the room next to theirs and she would just visit. But after I was born she never actually slept up there. My parents would tuck her into bed and the next morning they would find her wrapped in a blanket, sleeping in my room. There is a picture of Denise lying on the floor next to my crib, one arm wrapped around the wooden leg and the other holding my doll. She is almost a teenager in the photograph, but curled up on the shag carpet, she looks like a small child.

MY SISTER's hand is on the back of my neck. My body tenses up when she leans down and kisses the top of my head. I try to ignore her, but she gently turns my thin body over. She smooths the wrinkles on my bedspread and tells me it's not going to be that bad. Things will be different, but everything will be all right. She rubs her left temple and says I'm going to grow up to be a beautiful, smart, and responsible woman. She tells me I'm going to have a happy life. Even if the needles belong to me.

Mittens for the Diabetics

I DON'T GO TO the hospital right away. I cross my fingers that I'll be like one of the kids on television. I'll be able to avoid the needle too. But one day I hear my parents talking quietly in the kitchen. They think I'm in my bedroom playing, but I crouch between the cold wall and the couch in the living room and listen to their conversation. My mother says they have to watch me closely. My dad tells her not to worry. Magazines crumple under my feet as I shift my weight and press my ear to the wall. My mom says I'm too thin, my dad replies I've always been thin. I won't tell them the kids at school are telling me I look like a skeleton.

I have arguments with my best friend in the cafeteria about who weighs more, each of us wanting to be the heavier one. She always wins. She proves she's right by having the other kids compare us, asking them which one of us is thinner. She pulls me off the bench as I'm taking a sandwich out of my lunch box and leads me around the lunchroom, conducting her survey. The kids ask what's wrong with me—*isn't your mother feeding you?* They push the food they don't want from their sacks into my hand and tell me to go eat. They say I look like a starving child.

I know I'm not a starving child. The kids at school are stupid because a starving person doesn't have any food to eat. I understand how my body works. I have all the food I want, but my body just isn't turning all of it into energy. My dad does acidosis tests on me to make sure my body isn't feeding on itself. He sets a tiny white tablet on a white piece of paper and drops my urine onto the pill with an eyedropper. He says if it doesn't turn purple, we're okay. He picks up the piece of paper and studies the pill, comparing it to the color of the paper to see if it's changed. Acid will turn the pill a shade of purple if something is really wrong. My parents did these tests on my sister every week when she was little. Purple was the danger color. My pills are all staying white, so I don't care what the kids at school say. I'm not gaining any weight, but I'm not starving to death either.

WHILE MY dad scrapes ice off the windshield of his car, I curl up next to the heat vent in the living room every morning before school. I make a tent with a sheet and trap the warm air inside. My mom rolls her eyes and says I'm making the whole house cold. She says I act like I'm living in Siberia. I don't care. With my coat zipped up, I hold the sheet over my head and wait for my dad to come back inside and tell me the car is warm. One morning he walks in, drops his gloves on the carpet, and says we have to make a quick test. I'm irritated, but I push myself off the floor and go pee in the cup.

I sit on the edge of the bathtub and wait while he drops urine on the pill. His necktie dangles as he leans over the vanity. When he pulls the paper close to his face and examines it, I sit up taller. My boots dig into my backpack on the floor, and I strain my neck to see what he's looking at. He moves the pill to another section of the white paper with his fingernail. I wrap my fingers around the porcelain edge beneath me and push myself up. I tell him the pill is white, and I'm going to be late for school. He looks worried but drops the paper and the pill into the trash can.

The next day my mom tells my aunt we won't be going up to Minnesota for Christmas. She leans against the kitchen wall and presses the telephone receiver close to her mouth. She thinks I can't hear her. My parents don't want to take me that far from home, but I love going to my grandparents' farm in the winter. Endless fields of snow await where I can ride the snowmobiles and three-wheelers. My cousins will all be there, and the farmhouse is warm and smells like bread. I try to convince my parents I'm fine. I tell them that I don't think the pill looks purple in the least, but even if it is, it's not that big of a deal. They look at each other and tell me we can go visit my grandparents for only two days this year.

MY GRANDPARENTS meet us at the car on the snowy afternoon, two days before Christmas. My grandmother's alreadydrooping mouth drops more when she sees me. She narrows her eyes and hunches her 180-pound frame forward like she doesn't recognize me. We haven't been up to Minnesota since Easter, and I guess I look a lot different. She kisses me anyway and says she's going to feed me all weekend, but when I run off to play with the farm cats in the snow, my mother must explain the situation to her, because she doesn't give me anything sweet all weekend. She serves me potatoes and apples and healthy food. She bakes fresh peanut butter cookies for my cousins and an angel food cake for me. My brother walks out of the kitchen carrying four cookies, and I stare down at my own plate. A small white piece of cake. I know what it tastes like. My mother made my sister angel food cakes for her birthdays. Diabetic food. It tastes like a sponge. When my grandmother retreats to the living room, I drop the cake in the garbage and put the plate in the sink.

I grab my coat and boots from the hall closet. I want to go outside again. The heavy snow is perfect for a snowman. My boots are buckled and the thick scarf covers my cheeks and chin. I pull my purple stocking cap down over my ears and head for the front door. My grandmother steps in my path. I look down at myself. My hands aren't covered, and I take the mittens from my pockets and slip them on. I should have known I'd be caught for forgetting them. I start to step around her and she holds her arm out.

"Why don't you stay inside with me today?" she asks.

I look toward the door and back at her round face. She looks exactly like my mother but wrinkled.

"I'm gonna go build a snowman. I'll stay where you can see me. I'll be right by the porch." I raise my mitten toward the window.

She says it's too cold. She wants me to help her roll the yarn for a scarf. She's never asked me to roll yarn. I always play outside with my cousins.

"But I'm all bundled up," I reply.

She nods her head to confirm that I look ready to battle the harshest of Minnesota winters but raises her eyebrows to let me know there's no discussing it. My brother and two of my cousins tear through the house. Brian doesn't even look at me as he pulls open the front door and runs outside. He doesn't have his hat on, but my grandmother doesn't stop him. The cold air rushes in. My cousins follow my brother out, pulling the door closed behind them. I move my head to see out the window. They're throwing snow at each other and falling on their backs into the white flakes to make angels. I look back at my grandmother.

"Come on," she says, pulling the stocking cap from my head. "Let's go pick out a nice color."

I don't argue, but I'm going to tell my sister about this. She could talk my grandmother into letting me go outside. I look around the corner into the large room. All the adults are talking. They've brought in chairs from the dining room and sit facing each other. They do this every year. Denise is curled up on one end of the couch with a blanket wrapped around her shoulders. Her legs are tucked under her and she's laughing at something my uncle is telling her. He waves his hands around in the air as he talks. I try to catch her attention from the doorway, but she doesn't see me.

My grandmother has disappeared and I don't look for her. Instead I go back to the kitchen window and look outside. My brother has my cousin Danny down on the ground and he's pushing a snowball into his mouth. Brian sits on top of him while Danny tries to kick his legs up hard enough to push him off. Snow is coming down harder and my brother's black hair looks white. If I were out there, I would jump him from behind and rescue my cousin. Then Danny and I would gang up on him together and take him down.

"Crazy boys," a voice behind me says.

I don't turn around. I can see my grandfather's reflection looming over mine in the window. He's watching my brother and laughing. I hear my grandfather pull a plate from the cupboard and unwrap the angel food cake. He cuts himself a huge slice and heads back into the living room with the rest of the adults. I know he likes the cake. He has been diabetic forever, and a needle and a single bottle of insulin always sit on the corner of his oak dresser. I don't touch his needles though. I have played with my sister's at home but never my grandfather's. His are somehow different. Sacred.

My grandfather never talks about his diabetes. I've heard my mother talk about it though. She worries about her dad's health. She says that diabetes runs in our family. If one member of a family has diabetes, the chances are five times greater for other members to develop the disease. My grandfather, two of the cousins on my dad's side, and my sister all have it. Now I guess I do too.

I DON'T GET a box of chocolates on Christmas morning. My grandmother took it out from under the tree when I wasn't looking. She doesn't know I already examined all the packages with my name on them and recognized the familiar shake of Fanny Farmer chocolates. I end up with a new pair of mittens instead. I want to ask her what I'm going to do with a new pair of mittens when I can't go outside and play, but I keep my mouth shut because I know I'll get in trouble if I act ungrateful. My mom always tells us to pretend that we like whatever it is we unwrap, and we can complain about it in the car on the way home. I sit close to the tree and examine my presents. Denise bought me the makeup kit my mother said I was too young to have. I take the plastic tray from the box and smile up at my sister. She winks at me. I lock eyes with her and reach down and pick up the mittens. I hold them up near my face for her to see and wrinkle my nose. She smiles and shakes her head. There's a pair of mittens resting on top of her boxes too. I look around at everyone's presents. Fanny Farmer chocolates for the healthy people. Mittens for the diabetics.

In the middle of the night, I tiptoe down the creaking stairs and climb up onto the kitchen counter where my grandmother keeps her homemade cookies. Taking five from the jar, I quietly push the glass container back into its place and retreat to the guest room where I sleep with my cousins. None of them stir. Carefully I climb back into bed next to my brother and cram the cookies into my mouth. Crumbs fall onto the sheet between us. The granules of sugar get stuck between my teeth. My stomach feels satisfied for the first time in weeks. I don't feel guilty because no one has seen me. My brother is snoring softly and the house is quiet except for the usual, familiar creaks. I wipe my lips with the top of the bedspread before falling asleep.

Now THE purple on the white pills is obvious. I can't deny that the color is changing. It seems like all my dad does is examine my urine. My plastic cup rests next to the drain in the bathtub. I pull it from the tub, sit on the toilet, pee in it, and put it back in the tub. I can pee on demand now, even if it feels like there isn't a drop in my bladder. My mom told me to just close my eyes and completely relax my muscles. She says they only need a few drops. So I close my eyes, make my body go limp, and concentrate on peeing. Finally, a few drops trickle into the plastic cup in my hand.

My dad mixes drops with water in a test tube. We stare at it and wait. Blue then green and finally orange. Even though we know the colors and what they mean by heart, my dad always sets the color chart that comes with the bottle of tablets next to the test tube. He holds the little piece of paper up to the bottom of the tube and compares it. It's clearly orange, but he checks anyway. Sometimes the mixture runs the spectrum of colors slowly, and I cross my fingers that it stops on blue. And then green. But the bubbling solution taunts me, resting on blue for several seconds before zipping through the other colors to orange in the next few seconds. Then my dad fills the eye dropper up with my pee again and puts a drop on the little white pill. I pray that it will stay white, but it turns purple. He drops the sheet of paper into the trash and rinses the orange solution in the test tube down the drain. I look at the floor. He kisses the top of my head but says nothing. I know I have to go to the hospital soon.

THE SNOW IS heavy on my feet as I try to run through it. I fall down and make myself laugh out loud in front of the neighborhood kids. I tell my friend Blair I just tripped because I didn't get much sleep last night. The kids seize the opportunity to take the soccer ball from me. They've never been able to catch me before. I'm the best player on the block, but I'm getting too tired. I use all my energy to kick the ball far across the lawn before sitting down next to Blair's red hat. It marks the other team's goal. This is the first time I've left a game, and Blair follows me to the edge of the lawn.

"Move over that way," he yells at the kids on the lawn, motioning with one hand and forming a snowball with the other. "My mom doesn't think you look very good. She wants me to ask you if you're okay. She says she saw you fall off your bike or something, and you had trouble getting back on."

"Yeah, I hurt my knee. I'm fine now," I tell him.

We watch our friends playing. Blair throws his snowball at one of the boys, but no one notices. Too much snow is flying already. The neighborhood boys are moving farther away from us, and I look over at Blair. He's my only real friend on the street. The other kids are either my brother's age or several years younger than me. Blair and I stick together. He has lived two houses away from me ever since I was two.

"Well, I think I'm going to start giving shots like my sister," I say.

"Why?" he asks, narrowing his eyes.

I don't tell him that's a stupid question. I just say I have to go to the hospital.

"I'll come every day," he replies. "Maybe I can just come with you and I'll miss school too," he says.

I nod. I don't know much about how hospitals operate, but I don't think they'll let him stay with me. It's the first question I'm going to ask the nurse though.

He pulls his hands from his mittens and ties the laces on his boot. He doesn't look up at me when he speaks.

"My grandma has it too, and she's really healthy," he says. He goes on to talk about his grandmother, a diabetic woman in her sixties who still plays tennis three times a week. He tells me everyone in his family says she'll live to be a hundred.

I know there's a difference between juvenile-onset and later-onset diabetes, but I keep my mouth closed. My mom says adult diabetics don't get as sick as kids do. We drop lots of weight and become completely fatigued. And we're still growing, so it's harder to control our disease. I'm different from his grandmother, but I don't explain why. Blair won't listen anyway. He is a talker, and when I stand up to head home, he continues to talk. He walks me all the way to my front door with stories of his grandmother, but I'm not hearing him. My knees are weak and my mind is fuzzy. All the energy has drained out my body.

*　　　*　　　*

I TRACK SNOW through the kitchen. I know it will disappear before my parents get home from work; it's only 3:30. I open the basement door and listen for my brother. The light is on downstairs and I can hear him killing space invaders. He sits in front of the television with his Atari game every afternoon. Ignoring my mother when she calls him for dinner, he plays until my dad yells that he's going to come down and shut it off for him. Then my brother tries to eat his dinner quickly so he can get back to his game. My dad looks at the clock and looks at my brother shoveling food into his mouth and tells him that no matter how quickly he eats, he'll be sitting at the table for thirty minutes. I tell my brother that if he didn't act like he was in such a hurry, my dad wouldn't notice if he excused himself in twenty minutes. My dad says that Brian is just at that age where he has a lot of energy.

I sit down and look up at the telephone. I should call my mother at work and tell her I don't feel good. I know she'll come right home. My dad will make the drive home from downtown in half the normal time if I call him. I pick up a pen off the table and doodle on a coupon for chicken my mom cut out of the Sunday paper. She always tells me not to write on the coupons, but I draw a hat on the skinned chicken and give him back the face he lost when he was baked. I look at the clock again. I know my sister is probably at her house. Her afternoon classes are over and she studies at her kitchen table in the afternoons. I reach for the phone.

"Hello?" My sister sounds like she's been sleeping.

I open my mouth, but nothing comes out.

"Hello?" she asks again.

She'll think this is a prank phone call if I don't say something. Just as I'm about to hang up, I hear her voice.

"Andie? Is that you?"

"Uh-huh," I reply, wondering how she knows.

"You okay? What's wrong?" she asks.

"I'm okay," I say, looking down at the chicken on the coupon. I pick up the pen again and add stick legs and shoes. Silence.

"I think I'm ready to go," I tell her. I can hear her breathing. "I can't kick the soccer ball anymore, Dee Dee."

"I'll be over in a minute," she says, and I hear a click.

I hang up the phone and look down at my boots. They're dripping and I should take them off. Instead I track more melted snow through the living room and into my bedroom. I pull my suitcase from underneath my bed and open my dresser drawers. I pull a pink cardigan and jeans from my closet, carefully folding them into the suitcase. Then I throw in my clown, two books, my set of cooking pans, a deck of cards, and a package of Magic Markers. I can't get the lid zipped down, so I dig the jeans from the bottom of the pile and toss them on the bed. I push the clasps on the case down with my thumbs.

With snow from my stocking cap melting into my eyes and my hand wrapped around the handle of my suitcase, I stand in the doorway and look around my bedroom. I study it carefully, trying to memorize the way I'm leaving everything before I turn out the light. I know I'll be gone for a few weeks, and my brother will come in and steal my copies of *Mad* magazine. He'll hide them somewhere and tell my dad he doesn't know anything about it. I say good-bye to my dolls.

I sit on the edge of the living room couch and wait, straining my neck to look out the window every time a car goes by. I turn on the television and flip through the channels and turn it off. The house is silent except for an occasional cry from my brother downstairs as his tank gets shot by an alien invader. He doesn't know I'm up here. He thinks I'm still outside playing with the neighborhood kids. My coat is too warm and my feet are starting to sweat in my boots, but I stay dressed in my winter overclothes. The antique clock on the living room wall ticks.

My mother walks through the front door. Brushing

snowflakes off her coat, she sees me sitting on the edge of the couch clutching my suitcase. Her watery eyes stay frozen to the suitcase for several seconds. Usually she would pull off her fur-lined boots and hang her wet coat on the back of the door. Today she stays dressed and hovers in the doorway. I look back at the clock. She's home early. I know my sister called her.

"I called the hospital," she says.

I nod and look behind her to my sister. Denise is out of breath like she's been running. Snow is sticking to the bottoms of her jeans. I watch the snowflakes in her hair disappear. She stands too close to my mother. Finally she steps her snowy foot off the rug and onto the hardwood floor. My mother doesn't yell at her for it. Denise sits down on the couch next to me.

"So what happened today, Andie?" she asks.

"Nothing," I reply.

She nods and locks eyes with my mother.

"It's not going to be that bad," Denise says. She touches the ball on my stocking cap. "They're really nice people there. I was there too, ya know. You'll have a roommate and everything."

That's what I fear. They're going to put me in a room full of other diabetic kids and make us give shots to each other. I will become one of them. I'll have to ring a bell to go to the bathroom and they'll strap me to my bed at night. I've seen it all on television. And a roommate. I envision a deformed child limping on one leg from her bed to mine, telling me I have to feed her or read her a book. I'll probably have to take her to the bathroom in the middle of the night. Maybe she'll be dying and watch me with wild eyes all day. I'll have a needle hanging out of my leg and little kids will be running around me. My imagination starts to go crazy and my sister sees it on my face.

"It'll be okay there," she says.

I try to believe her, but she might be saying this because my mother is listening. She always tells me the truth, but she tells it to me when we're alone. When my cousin died and no one would talk to me about it, Denise explained what death meant.

She took me outside the church and said his body didn't work anymore. It would happen to all of us eventually. Even her someday, she said. She talks to me about everything, not just the kid stuff. I can ask her stupid questions and I know she'll answer me. But sometimes she gets less honest when my parents are around. I look up at my mother. She's leaning against the orange plaid chair and staring at the wall. I think she's going to start crying, so I look at Denise. She raises her eyebrows and I know she's telling me the truth about the hospital. She's been there enough. She wouldn't lie to me about it.

"You ready?" my sister asks, forcing a thin smile.

I hesitate and a hundred reasons not to go fill my head. I feel much better. I could go out and play ball with Blair now. I can go take a nap and I'll wake up refreshed. My head isn't spinning and I can hear the kids yelling in the yard next door. I know I could postpone the hospital visit one more day, but I nod to my sister.

"Come on, you can ride in front with me," Denise says. She picks up my suitcase and stands.

The three of us walk single file out to my sister's silver Camaro. My mom climbs in the backseat and tells me to fasten my seat belt. Denise turns the radio up and hums the whole way to downtown Des Moines. I look at the people in the skywalks. Men in business suits are rushing home to their families. My sister drives slowly through the snow-covered streets. None of us speak.

Getting Tagged

THE NURSE'S red hair and pink blouse clash with the mustard-yellow walls in my room. Her mouth is big and she doesn't have any eyelashes. She flashes me a huge smile and asks me if I go by the name Andrea. I lean against the doorway and say nothing. The room smells too clean, like no one has ever really slept here. I know I have a roommate because there are two beds. My sister is unpacking my suitcase and my mother is sitting on a plastic orange chair. Forms are stacked on her lap. She scratches her forehead with the plastic hospital pen.

The nurse moves closer to me, cocking her head to the left, waiting for me to speak. I scratch my arm through my thick winter coat but keep quiet. The woman gives me a satisfied nod anyway and spreads a white gown with blue flowers across a chair. It's paper thin from too many washes. There are snaps up the back and the material is frayed around the edges. I open my eyes wide and stare at my mother.

"Just for tonight," my mom says, nodding toward the thin gown. "I'll bring your pajamas tomorrow."

"Oh, that's okay," the nurse begins. Her voice is too cheery. "It would be best if she just wore our gowns while she's here. We'll be sure she has a clean one every day." She straightens her earring and smiles at me again. "We'll just stick with the program."

My mom raises her eyebrows and taps her pen against the clipboard stacked with forms. This is the same look she gets when my brother does something stupid. Her mouth starts to open like she's going to yell at this woman, but she exhales loudly instead.

"I'll bring them tomorrow," she says flatly, and looks back down at the forms.

That's the final word and the nurse knows it. The smile on her face disappears. My mother has this way of intimidating people into shutting up. It's the way she looks at them with her eyebrows arched and her lips pursed. I've heard the stories about how she argued with my sister's doctors when Denise was growing up. My sister told me our mother used to start every sentence with the words, "I've had a diabetic kid longer than you've been practicing medicine, and . . ." If my mom didn't like the instructions a doctor gave, she argued until he agreed to do it her way. She knows more about diabetes than anyone I know, but I'm relieved she didn't yell at the nurse. I have to stay here by myself with these people tonight.

The pink nurse asks to take my coat. I have no intention of moving. She pulls a plastic wristband and a pair of scissors from her large pocket. She's going to tag me. Not even my mother can save me from this, so I slowly unzip my coat and take a step into the room. A mitten falls out of the pocket and I take my time picking it up. I've seen the way it irritates my mother when she tells me to do something and I move in slow motion. I pull my arms out of the jacket one at a time and place it on the chair, completely covering the white gown. The woman runs her fingers over the sleeve and tells me it sure does look warm. Her nails are bright pink.

"We'll just put this around your wrist here," the nurse says. She kneels down in front of me and I can see down her shirt. Her chest is covered with freckles. She holds the plastic strip out and waits for me to give her my arm. I turn away and look down at my boots. Then I bend over to pull them off. Slowly.

They're dripping and I kick them under the bed. My white socks are hanging off the ends of my feet.

"I'll just put this on your wrist, honey," she says, moving the strip back and forth to the rhythm of her words. She looks like a duck sitting on her feet moving toward me.

Finally, I hold my arm straight out. She wraps the band around my wrist and cuts the excess plastic off with the scissors in one snip. I bring my wrist up to my face. My name and social security have been typed perfectly across the band. I'm official.

The woman's knees crack as she stands up and takes a step back. It crosses my mind to hold my arm above my head and scream that the band is cutting off my circulation. I've seen criminals on television go into rages about their handcuffs being too tight. Sometimes the cops loosen them and sometimes they tell the robbers to shut up. I suspect this woman would just smile, so I don't say anything.

She goes on to tell us that visiting hours will be over in fifty minutes. My roommate will be back shortly and an orderly will be in to draw blood. I want to ask what an orderly is, but my mother and sister aren't talking to her, so I don't either. I find out soon enough anyway.

A man in white walks in and nods at me. He sets his plastic tray on the nightstand and pats the side of the bed. His hands are dark and hairy. There's no point looking to my mother or sister for help. Denise has pulled another plastic chair up next to my mother, and they're looking through a folder the nurse gave them. I sit down on the bed and watch the man. He pulls a huge syringe and short rubber tube from the tray. The syringe has the longest needle I've ever seen, and it fascinates me for a moment. Then he reaches for my arm. I want to tell him the needle won't fit in there, but he wraps the tubing around my biceps. Now I do feel like screaming that my circulation is being cut off, but I stay quiet. He's slapping the inside of my arm with two of his hairy fingers. I squeeze my eyes shut just as the needle pushes through the surface of my skin. My shoulders are tense and I wait for more pain, but I can't feel anything. When I open my eyes, I see that the needle has disappeared into my arm. My blood flows easily into the tube. Pulsing through the needle to the beat of my heart. He pulls the needle out, puts a cotton ball over the spot, bends my arm, and walks back out of the room as quietly as he entered.

THAT WAS my first donation. And it was the easiest. The next day the orderly discovers that he can't find a vein to poke in my other arm. He slaps his fuzzy fingers around for several minutes and finally tells me the vessels won't cooperate. He's sorry, but he has to use the same spot again. And again. Four times a day an orderly comes to collect my blood, and I hate them all. I wander around in the halls when I know they're coming. I make them track me down. When they do catch me and bring me back to my room, I open my arm out onto the bed, never looking up at them. The inside of my right arm is black and blue. I can't bend it anymore.

My roommate has it worse than I do. Cancer is growing in her leg. The nurses come in the morning to give her shots. She starts to cry the moment they appear, and I can hear her moan when they push the needle in. Every sound slips through the white curtain between us, but the nurses always pull it shut anyway. When my roommate goes away for treatments in the afternoon, she comes back and takes a nap. She touches her head and says that more of her hair will fall out now. She walks with a limp and doesn't snore. Her name is Jessica and she's a year younger than me. I like her. When she laughs, her whole body shakes.

We play with the other kids on the floor. We pretend the two-year-old boy down the hall is our son, and we build a house out of huge blocks. Brad is here because his mother wrapped a rubber band around his thumb when he wouldn't stop sucking it. She left it on for two days and then got scared when it turned purple, finally deciding to take him to the doctor. My mom says they're keeping him here because there's nowhere else to put him. One of the older kids told Jessica that the doctors are going to cut the thumb off. It's black and looks dead, but Jessica and I believe we can nurse him back to health. We make him a bed out of pillows and prepare him lunch.

Mostly I play between visits from the orderlies and doctors. I have to pee for the nurses a lot, and they ask me stupid questions like whether or not I'm sneaking candy from the other kids. They don't have any candy, I reply. But they're not diabetic. None of them. These kids are here for surgeries and cancer and heart problems. My illness is simple compared to theirs. As soon as I start giving myself shots, I'll be able to go back home. Some of these kids have been here for weeks. I tell Jessica I'll be leaving soon and if she just had diabetes instead of cancer she could get out of here too. When she asks me what diabetes is, I try to explain it to her.

"If your pancreas," I say, pointing to her lower abdomen, "didn't work, you would have diabetes. It's when the cells aren't making any insulin. Then there's sugar in your pee and your body can't use any of the food you're eating."

"That's why you're so skinny?" she asks.

I nod. She is skinny too, but I know I shouldn't tell her. I think she's even skinnier than me.

"So if someone shot a hole through my stomach and hit my pancreas, it would make it so I had to give shots?" she asks.

I think about her question. Yesterday I told her that I'm going to be giving my own shots soon, and she's fascinated.

"I don't think so," I tell her. "It's the cells. I guess if they shoot holes in all the cells, you'd have to." I'm not sure. My sister probably knows.

Jessica stares at me, thinking about what I've said, and finally nods like she understands. Then she explains the cancer in her leg.

I have never known anyone with cancer. My mother talks about people at work who get it, but I've never really listened.

Jessica explains that her body is working against her. She says that bad cells are multiplying and the doctors are killing them. She tells me she heard the doctor talking to her mother about not being able to get them all. She stares across the room at Brad's hand and talks about maybe having to get a new leg. She compares it to Captain Hook in *Peter Pan,* and I wonder why the doctors can't just get me a new pancreas.

Jessica and I are different from the other kids on our floor. We understand what's wrong with our bodies. Some of the kids, even the older ones, can't give us a reason for why they're in the hospital. They know it has something to do with their heart or kidneys, but they just shrug when we ask them what exactly is wrong. No one has explained anything to them. My mom tells me everything about what's going on here, even if she knows it's going to make me cry. She has taken a vacation from work and stays in my room all day, asking the doctors a lot of questions when they come to see me.

When I go to the playroom, my mom sits in the orange plastic chair and talks to Jessica's mom. Sometimes I sneak back to my room and listen to the conversations from the hallway. I sit with my back pressed against the door and smile at the nurses when they walk by. Jessica's mom talks about her divorce and raising Jessica by herself. My mom talks about her job and Denise's college. It's grown-up conversation and it gets boring fast, but sometimes I hear things I'm not supposed to be hearing. Jessica's dad hit her mom and pulled the phone out of the wall in their apartment before the divorce. My mom's voice shakes when she talks about my dad's office reorganizing. Sometimes they lower their voices and speak too softly, like they know I'm sitting just outside. I head back down the hall to the playroom.

Most of the kids are younger than I am, and they brag a lot. The boy getting heart surgery says his family is moving to Disneyland when he gets out. I tell him he's lying. Real people don't live in Disneyland. But he shrugs like he doesn't care if I believe him or not. Another one of the boys says he has seven bicycles at home, one for each day of the week. I miss my regular friends. They might exaggerate, but they don't lie like this. My mom says these kids stray from the truth because they're trying to impress each other. She says they're lonely. And most of the kids are here all alone. Two of the kids across the hall from my room never have any visitors.

"Where could his mother be?" my mom asks my dad. "Even if his parents work, you'd think they would still come in the evening. Don't you, Ray?" She rolls her eyes at my father and says, "I can't believe that little boy never has anyone in to see him."

My dad shrugs and tells her he doesn't understand either. He comes to see me every day after work. The hospital is only a few minutes from his office, and he walks in wearing a sport coat and shiny black shoes. He looks important and I know he's going to stay through dinner. Jessica's father comes only on Saturdays and doesn't like to play games. My dad stays until visiting hours are over and plays with Jessica too. I think those kids whose parents don't come are going to die. Die alone. I have nightmares about the nurses wheeling their bodies out while we sleep at night.

JESSICA always falls asleep before I do. When the nurses pull the curtain closed between us and turn the lights off, we talk about what we're going to do the next day. We talk about going back to school and which nurse is our favorite. Then she just stops talking, sometimes right in the middle of a story. I ask her if she's sleeping, and there's no response. I look over at the long white curtain before turning onto my stomach. I wiggle my hands under my belly and fall asleep.

Sometimes I wake up in the middle of the night. The nurses have pushed the bars up on the side of my bed and the room is quiet. I look over at the white curtain. Every night Jessica asks the nurses to leave it open, but they just smile and pull it closed anyway. The window is on her side, but light from the hallway comes in through the crack under the door. Occasionally, a nurse walks by or a telephone rings, but mostly it's just quiet. My parents are home sleeping, but if they were here they would sit with me until I fall back asleep. The only telephone I could use to call them is down the hall behind the counter, but the nurse wouldn't let me anyway. My eyes dart around the room and my chest feels tight. I want to run for the bathroom and flip on the light, but I can't figure out how to work the bars. I close my eyes and listen to Jessica breathe.

A NURSE wakes me up early every morning. The room is still too dark to make out which one of the women is standing over me. When my eyes finally adjust, I see the small metal tray. I recognize the syringe and the vials of insulin. She tells me to push up the sleeve of my pajamas while she pulls an alcohol swab from a plastic package. She holds it between her thumb and index finger and waits for me to move. I don't. Instead I pick the needle up off the tray and pull off the orange cap. She takes the needle from my hand and asks me again to roll up my sleeve. I'm fully awake now and try to convince her that I'm an expert with the needles, but she won't believe me. She won't believe I know how to give a shot. Going through what I will soon learn to be the standard procedure, she inserts the needle into the back of my left arm. She looked at the right one first, but didn't want to touch it because of the big bruise where they take my blood. She pokes it in and out quickly, and it doesn't hurt as much as I always thought it would.

She leaves the room and returns carrying a bigger silver tray with an orange, alcohol swabs, a bottle of insulin, and six needles. Daylight streams through the window now, and she tells me to practice giving shots to the orange. I look up at her like she's stupid, but she eases the tray onto my lap. Then she sits on the side of the bed and watches me. I pick the bright orb up and examine it. It's a perfect piece of fruit, and I tell her that oranges are for eating, not injecting. She's not impressed. So I pull liquid into the syringe, set the orange on the sheet covering my legs, and swab the surface. The smell of alcohol makes my nose burn. I stick the needle through the tough skin and push the plunger down. She seems satisfied, but she makes me do it again. Practice makes perfect, she says. When she leaves me alone for a moment, I peel the orange and rip it into slices. I arrange them on the tray around the needles and wait for her to return. She says nothing, picks up the sloppy tray, and returns with a new piece of fruit, sitting on my bed until I have correctly administered ten shots.

WITH MY first insulin shots come my first insulin reactions. Jessica and I are sprawled on the floor of our room putting together a jigsaw puzzle. Before my mom went to lunch, she propped the lid of the box up against the wall, reminding us to look at it if we needed to. It is a picture of two covered bridges in the country. The sky is bright and the grass is tall and green. We're each doing our own corner, trading pieces and snapping the funny shapes in place. It's the hardest puzzle I've ever put together. There are 200 pieces and they all look the same. We've sorted them into piles by color, but one bit of grass looks just like the next. I'm looking from the box to the pile of brown pieces when my vision starts to blur. I focus my eyes on the picture and stare at the wooden bridge. Jessica is turning a piece over in her hand and telling me about the bike her dad is buying her for her birthday. She says it's blue and the best one in the store. I rub my eyes and try to blink the haze away.

The skin on my stomach crawls, and I push myself up onto my butt and cross my legs. I look down at the pieces and spot the one I've been looking for. My hand shakes as I pick it up. I'm getting scared. My breathing is uneven and my heart is racing, but I keep staring at the puzzle.

"What are you doing?" Jessica asks.

I hear her voice through a fog. I bend down and put my head between my knees. My brother does this when he has a bloody nose, and I wonder if it will work for my dizziness. Once I've closed my eyes, I can't open them. I think about how Denise describes her insulin reactions. She says she gets weak and shaky when there's too much insulin in her body. The first day I was here, she told me I should expect them too and left some candy in my nightstand. The nurses don't know it's there, but I know I have to eat it.

I stand up and steady myself by leaning against the wall. Jessica is looking at the door like she should go get some help. I pull the peppermint pinwheels from the drawer and put three of them in my mouth.

"You're not supposed to eat those," she informs me.

I want to tell her that it's different now, but my mouth is full of candy and I don't think I have the energy to speak anyway.

"I'm calling Marsha," Jessica says, pushing the red button over my bed. It's the first time she has called the nurse by her real name. Jessica's mom referred to the woman in pink as "Nurse Ratched," and we don't know what it means, but that's what we call her too.

Another nurse comes rushing in, takes one look at my face swelled with candy, and holds her hand under my chin. I don't know what else to do, so I spit the pinwheels out. She asks what I'm doing, but I just close my eyes.

Then the technician appears in the doorway and whispers something to the nurse. He moves toward me quickly. I barely feel the prick of the needle. The nurse returns holding a glass of orange juice. She presses it to my lips, and the taste of mint in my mouth makes the juice bitter. I drink it anyway, because now the nurse looks sorry.

By the time my mother gets back, I feel fine. I want to tell her that the nurse took my candy, but I don't say anything. Jessica doesn't either. I told her to keep quiet. We stay on the floor and work on the puzzle. It's almost half done and it looks just like the picture on the box. If I tell my mom, she'll walk down the hall and ask the nurses for the whole story. She doesn't need to know about the funny feeling anyway. This happens to my sister all the time, and she just slips a piece of candy in her mouth and goes back to whatever she's doing. She doesn't make a big deal out of it.

I KNOW when the funny feeling is coming. It's a good thing too, because it seems to take the nurses forever to get me any juice. They never believe me when I tell them my blood sugar is getting low. They go back down the hall to their desk and call the technician. I watch the clock on my nightstand. I have to wait for orange juice while the hairy man takes the blood down to the lab and calls the nurse to tell her the reading. I know when the phone rings, she'll be in with the juice.

The candy in my nightstand disappears. When I ask Jessica if she ate it, she tells me the nurse in pink put it all in her pocket and walked out of the room shaking her head. I know they don't believe me about the insulin reactions because they think I just want some candy. Sometimes when I tell them the funny feeling is coming, they ask me if I'm sure. They ask if I ate some candy. I want to tell them that if I'd eaten the candy, I wouldn't be standing in front of their desk asking for juice. But I look at the wall and shake my head. Finally, they pick up the phone and call the hairy man.

When I wake up with insulin reactions in the middle of the night, I have to ring the bell. I still haven't figured out how to work the bars on the side of my bed. The nurse wanders into my room and tells me I'll have to wait for a technician. The man on duty takes forever when it's late at night. I wait a long time, usually falling back asleep, hoping they don't forget about me. I'm too weak to get mad, and I know they don't understand how I feel. My back sinks into the mattress and my arms tingle. Finally, a nurse shakes my shoulder and presses a plastic glass to my lips. I tell my mom the next morning.

Her eyes get wide, and she turns her back to me and marches out of the room. I jump up and peek around the corner after her. She is stomping down the hall. The nurse behind the counter stands up. My mother raises her voice, and I can hear her perfectly as she informs the woman that nothing like this had better happen ever again. If her daughter says her blood sugar is low, it's low. She tells the woman to leave the candy in my nightstand or there's going to be trouble. I know about trouble with my mom, and the nurse acts like she does too. I can hear the woman apologizing. She says something to my mom about standard procedure, but my mom turns her back on the woman and raises her hand like she's not listening. The people in the hospital listen to my mother.

The Circle

THEY WON'T let me give my shots until I finish classes on managing diabetes. The nurses tell me they're mandatory. When I give them a blank stare, they explain that means I have to attend. I try to convince my dad I already know everything about diabetes, and it would probably even save him some money if I didn't go. My mom's requested a copy of the hospital charges up until now and complained to my dad. It was six pages long and my mom said she couldn't believe they charged fifty cents for two aspirin tablets. She called the hospital a rip-off joint. They make my parents pay for every little thing, even the needles I use on the oranges. I tell my dad we should just go home, but he says the classes are free and I have to attend.

I take the elevator by myself to the third floor. An old nurse in a white dress and black hose meets me at the door. She's the only nurse I've seen with a name tag. Claire. I look past her into the room. No kids. Four men and one woman sitting in a circle stare back at me like I'm in the wrong place. I think so too. Even though there are no other diabetic kids in the pediatrics ward with me, I somehow expected them to be here. But the people in this classroom look older than my parents. They probably have grandchildren my age. I start to turn around and the nurse says my name. I stare at the bump on her nose, and she points to a seat next to another old woman. Claire tells me to join the circle.

"So, have you all been giving your own shots by now?" the nurse asks.

I shake my head and everyone else nods.

"Anyone have any questions about the procedure yet?" she asks.

The man across the circle speaks up.

"Is it really necessary to swab the skin after the injection? My brother has been giving shots for years and I've never seen him do it," he says.

"Ah, yes. Important to reduce the chances of infection. Let me just go through exactly what administering an injection entails." Claire passes out sheets with a list of the steps for giving a shot and begins reading them out loud.

"First, make sure the insulin you're using is completely mixed in the vial. For those of you using NPH or any of the Lente, you must roll the bottle in your hands several times before you draw insulin. If you don't do this, it will either be too potent or too weak," she informs us, looking up to see if we're following along on the paper.

"Next wash the site of the injection with soap and water and apply alcohol with a cotton swab."

I roll my eyes and settle back into my chair. Claire stops to explain the peak times for insulin. Regular insulin acts quickly. NPH in about four hours. Lente takes even longer to peak. I know all this, so I study the woman sitting next to me. She is wearing a hospital gown and her graying hair is rolled in pink sponge curlers. Listening carefully with her eyes narrowed, she plants her fuzzy slippers firmly on the linoleum and moves her head in the direction of Claire. She's acting like the kids at school who try to kiss up to the teachers. They pretend to pay attention and point to the book when they're asking questions. Those kids always annoy the rest of the class, but I feel sorry for this woman next to me. Deep wrinkles surround her eyes. She looks like she's really listening.

"So," Claire continues, raising her voice and staring at me, "you set the plunger of your syringe at the mark of your dosage and stick the needle into the rubber stopper on the vial. Push the air into the bottle. Pull the plunger back to the mark showing your dosage. If there are air bubbles, push the insulin back in or tap the syringe with your finger."

I watch her now. She is demonstrating with a real syringe, and I spot the bowl of oranges on the table next to her. I know what's coming. We're going to practice on more fruit, like a quiz to see if we've been listening. I focus my attention on what she's doing so I don't have to stay after class and practice.

My sister never uses soap or alcohol. If she runs out of needles, she digs a syringe out of the garbage and uses it again. My sister calls the information about germs a scare tactic. She says it was created by people trying to sell more prescriptions for syringes. They're making us think giving a shot is supposed to be a major medical procedure. She says she can't contaminate her own body, and sometimes she uses the same syringe four or five times.

"Now," Claire says, picking up one of the oranges, "hold the needle steady and inject it into the site quickly and deeply, at a ninety-degree angle."

She stabs the needle into the fruit, and one of the men shudders and looks away. A giggle escapes from my throat, but I immediately close my mouth and stare down at the sheet of paper in my hand. Claire snaps her head in my direction.

"Remember, once the needle is in place you have to pull the plunger back and check the syringe for blood. If you ever get blood in your syringe, you'll know you've hit a capillary and you need to start all over. Pull the needle out immediately and start over. You can't inject insulin directly into the bloodstream. Not only will it shock your system with insulin, resulting in an immediate insulin reaction, but if there's an air bubble in there that you didn't get out, we could be in real trouble." Claire holds the orange up and pushes the plunger down.

My eyes drift away from the nurse, and I spot my mom looking through the square of glass on the door. Her face is framed in the window like a photograph hanging on a wall. She is staring at the orange in Claire's hand. I move the plastic ID tag on my wrist and look at my watch. One hour a day for eight days and Claire tells us we'll learn all about diabetes. Everything we need to know to live a normal, healthy life, she says. When she looks up at the clock on the wall behind me, her pace quickens. She passes out the oranges, syringes, and swabs, telling us to practice a few times on the fruit. I think I might be able to slip out of the room, but the woman next to me starts asking questions. She wonders why we can't just take some kind of insulin pill.

"It just doesn't work like that," Claire replies.

The woman asks why.

"The body can't use insulin unless it enters through the tissues. That makes the body believe it really came from the cells in your own pancreas." She pulls her lips together tightly and shakes her head, satisfied that she's answered the woman's question.

I could explain it to the woman in curlers, but I don't want to speak. The juices in her stomach would destroy the insulin. People have tried swallowing insulin. It doesn't work. My parents have been reading the articles on breakthroughs in diabetes since my sister was little, and there's no other way to get the hormone into the body. Scientists have tried nose sprays and pills. There's no choice. I give two perfect injections to the orange, slip my shoes back on, and walk toward the door to my mother.

"How'd it go?" she asks.

"I'm not going back," I reply. "I don't like that woman and everyone in there is old."

"It's only a few days, Andie. It's not going to kill you." I begin to say that I have to go to the class for eight more days and

I've already been in the hospital six, but she looks like she's going to cry, so I keep quiet. She puts her arm around my shoulder and pushes the button by the elevator.

We have a book at home written in the sixties by a doctor who worked with diabetic kids. My mom says it was the only book she could find that related to my parents and Denise back then. It says that when a kid gets diabetes, the doctor has two patients. The mother and the child. My mom worries about me. She tries not to show it, but I know she worries about the rest of my life. The same way she still worries about my sister. I lean into her side and put my arm around her waist as we wait for the elevator.

THE NEXT day I take the elevator for a ride. I stop on every floor, pushing the Open Door button and sticking my head out into the hallways. They all look the same. A plant and mirror greet me as soon as the door opens. When doctors and nurses get on, I step to the back of the elevator and push the plastic ID bracelet up under my sleeve. They glance at me like they're going to say something but turn and face the door instead. When people in street clothes carrying flowers or balloons step on the elevator, I ask them what floor they're headed to. I push the button. They smile down at me and tell me the floor number. None of them go to the pediatrics ward.

A harried woman in a black leather coat gets on. I go through the routine of welcoming her to the elevator and asking for her floor. My index finger hovers around the buttons. She tells me to push number two. My floor. Then she looks at me suspiciously and asks where I'm heading. Just visiting my mom, I tell her, up on the seventh floor. I point my finger into the air and smile. She asks what's wrong with my mother. I think for a second about launching into a story about cancer. Jessica has filled me in on all the procedures. But I don't have to answer. The elevator beeps and the woman steps off. I press my back against the wall in case any of my nurses are walking by. Then I push number five and head for my class.

I'm almost fifteen minutes late, but Claire doesn't look at me like I'm in trouble. Instead she extends her arm and welcomes me into the room. I take my place in the circle. She's handing out Medic Alert bracelets and ID cards. She pulls a special bracelet out for me. It's a smaller version of the bright silver ones she gave to everyone else. She tells me to put it on, and I look down at the plastic strip already secured around my wrist. Water has seeped underneath the plastic and smudged the letters of my name. The edges are getting frayed. I put the silver bracelet in my pocket.

The card has blanks to write my name and address. It says: "I am a diabetic. If I am unconscious or behaving abnormally I may be having an insulin reaction. If I can swallow, give me sugar, candy, fruit juice, or a sweetened drink. If I cannot swallow, send me immediately to the hospital." I'm not sure what to do with the card, so I put it in my pocket too. When I look up, everyone is studying them. They've all put the bracelets on, and they keep running their fingers over them, twisting them around on their wrists. I pull the sleeves of my sweater down over my hands, and Claire starts talking.

She talks the whole hour. She tells us diabetes is the leading cause of blindness and amputation. She says it contributes to high blood pressure and heart disease and it's the fourth leading killer in the U.S. She talks about how we should be washing our feet and going to the doctor every three months. I stare at the clock on the wall, counting the minutes until I can go. She knows I'm not paying attention and after class she asks me where my bracelet is. I pull it from my pocket and she says I can put it on.

I stare down at the little metal band.

"You need to keep it on your wrist at all times, and put the card in your schoolbag," she informs me.

I look around the empty classroom.

"You're kidding, right?" I ask.

I'm not going to wear the bracelet. The kids at school will ask me questions. They'll want to know what the red symbol means. I've heard the stories about how kids used to tease my sister for being diabetic. I've seen the way the boys a grade ahead of me tease the epileptic kid. They walk up to him at recess and drop to the ground, pretending to shake uncontrollably. The kid cries and runs inside to tell the teacher. I'm going to throw the bracelet away when I get back to my room.

"Andie," she sighs, "I don't like this any better than you do, but you have to just accept it. The bracelet is there to save your life." She pauses and studies my face. "It isn't fair for a pretty little eight-year-old to go through this."

"Nine," I reply, staring into her eyes. "I'm nine. And I'm not just going to keel over and die in the middle of the playground at school." I wrap my fingers tightly around the metal, trying to crush it.

She doesn't know how to respond, so she turns around and starts to gather up her books. I push open the door and head for the stairs. I'm not going to ride on the elevator with Claire.

MY FINGERS don't even shake a bit when I grasp the syringe between them. I can feel the nurse staring at me as I draw the insulin from the vial and replace the orange cap. Two units of Regular insulin, one unit of NPH. There's room for fifty units in the syringe, so it looks like only a few drops through the clear plastic tube. I swab the skin with alcohol and glance up at her. She nods in approval. My sister calls this playing the hospital game. Denise tells me to do what the doctors and nurses ask while I'm here. I hold the syringe at a 90-degree angle and push the needle into the skin on the back of my left arm. Just a little sting. My skin is soft, and there's no resistance to the needle. The metal tip disappears beneath the surface of my skin, and I pull back the plunger to check the syringe for blood. My muscle tightens and expands in response to the insulin.

THE NURSES are still asking me if I'm eating candy. I don't even answer them anymore. They say my blood sugars are too high in the morning and too low at night. They adjust my insulin, monitor my food, keep track of my activity. Trial and error. Nothing works. My mom argues with them in the hallway. I hear the doctor say I can't leave until everything is stabilized, and my mother tells him that I need to be at home to get me on a real schedule. All I do is pee in the cup and give them my blood. It's not enough. So I tell the nurse I can't pee anymore. I take the cup into the bathroom and sit on the edge of the bath-tub for five minutes before opening the door. The floor is spot-less and the shower curtain is wet. Then I open the door, hand the nurse the empty cup, and say I just can't do it. She gives me a glass of water and tells me she'll wait. I need my sister.

I'M SITTING on the edge of my bed waiting for Denise when she walks in. Her fingers are wrapped around a new Judy Blume book, and her long leather coat hangs over her shoulders. Her eyes light up when she sees me.

"How ya doing?" she asks, looking around the room and putting the book on my nightstand.

I force a smile and tell her to sit in the chair.

"I was thinking of a way to get me out of here faster," I say. I've been rehearsing this conversation in front of the bathroom mirror, but now my heart is racing.

She raises her eyebrows and waits for me to continue.

"Well, they're not gonna let me out of here because my blood sugars are too high. I thought maybe you could pee in this cup," I said, pulling the cup I had been saving from the drawer. "You could leave it for me to use instead of my own. Then they'll let me come back home."

"Andie," she sighs, shaking her head. "You're being silly. They've got your blood work four times a day too. They would know it's not your urine. And besides, my urine has sugar in it too. Why are they still high?"

I just stare at her.

"Are you sneaking candy from the other kids?" she asks.

I slowly shake my head. The sun is setting. The huge ball is right outside the window, and even though it's covered by a haze, it burns my eyes.

"They'll get regulated pretty soon. It doesn't take them long. Just a few more days to balance everything out and then they'll let you go. Cheating them doesn't really help you, you know."

I know.

Denise sighs again and her eyes roam across my face. Then she smiles.

"Pretty clever though," she says. "You're always thinking. But you know it's going to be over soon. The doctors just want to be sure you're healthy and okay before they send you home. Otherwise, you're no better when you leave than when you came in."

I'm not trying to be clever. I'm sick of it here. I even miss my brother.

"Well, maybe Jessica can pee for me then," I say. "She has cancer in her leg, but her pancreas is working."

My sister rubs her forehead. Her knuckles look dry.

"That's not the point, Andie. And you know it. You'd never get away with it anyway, and even though you think you might want to, you really don't. Just a few more days."

So I pee in the nurse's cup. My sister is right. The next day, all my urine tests and blood work come back okay. One more day of class and I can go home. I've gained twelve pounds. When my dad tells me the doctor is going to sign the release, I hold out my hand for him to slap. He smiles and lightly smacks his palm against mine. I go to the playroom to tell the kids I'm leaving.

*   *   *

MY PARENTS attend my last management class with me. Friday is family and friend day, and the extra people make the circle seem too big. Claire spends the entire hour talking again.

"It all might be very hard to accept right now. Diabetes can be lived with and maintained, but you might feel depression for a time. It is normal and will pass. It may seem like people treat you differently now, as if you're sick. Let them know that you're happy. Healthy." She smiles.

I want to tell my parents that the nurse never smiles this much when they aren't here. I nudge my mom and roll my eyes, but she keeps staring at the woman. My father is holding her hand.

"And you might feel like rebelling at first," Claire continues. "Against the advice of your physician or even the disease itself. It's not uncommon to feel that way. Just remember, when you rebel, you increase your chances of insulin reactions and ketosis. Talk to your primary physician about how you feel. Find a productive way to deal with your aggressions."

I look around the room. I know everyone's name now. James and Ted are with their wives, and Betty, who I've still never seen without curlers in her hair, is sitting next to her daughter. She looks even older today. Thomas and Ernie are alone. Tom has been divorced almost ten years, and Ernie's wife died a few months ago. Claire told us stress can trigger diabetes that may have been dormant for years.

"Your loved ones will have trouble differentiating between your normal mood swings and those related to your fluctuating blood sugars," Claire says. "Be patient with each other. Understand that this is the family's disease to live with too. Diabetic relatives might even feel guilt," she says, glancing at me.

No one asks any questions when Claire finishes talking, but they wander around the room like they're lost. I pull on my dad's shirtsleeve. He holds up his finger for me to wait and goes to the front of the room to talk to Claire. He's thanking her. I know she's wishing him good luck with me. They all think I'm just being difficult. I'm not. I just want my dad to stay on my side, so I approach them and take his hand. He looks down at me, puts one arm around my shoulder, and extends the other to Claire. They shake hands for only a second before I pull him toward the door.

I DROP MY suitcase on the braided rug in the living room and slip the boots off my feet. My socks slide on the hardwood floor as I run to my bedroom. Everything is exactly as I left it, but it seems like I've been away for years. I stare at my miniature kitchen appliances in disgust. I envision posters of rock stars and athletes taped to the walls, replacing the framed pictures of the characters from Winnie the Pooh. There are too many stuffed animals covering my bed, and I'm suddenly ashamed of the Barbie dolls in a heap on the floor. Picture books from my childhood line the shelves. Lowering myself onto the pastel bedspread, I hear the rumple of paper in the pocket of my jeans. Jessica's phone number is scribbled on white notebook paper.

Ripping at the edges of the little sheet, I walk to the bookshelf and count my comic books. Brian has taken two. I pull them all off the shelf and spread them out on the floor, trying to figure out exactly which ones are missing. There were seventeen of them two weeks ago, but now I'm not sure which two are gone. I won't get them back anyway. He's put them somewhere I won't find them, and he'll say he doesn't know what I'm talking about.

My father walks in and sets my suitcase on the bed. It's an ugly plastic box that says "Going to Grandma's." I'm going to ask for a new one. The sticker of the cartoon kid is peeling off and one of the clasps is broken. It's too small for me now. My clothes are getting too big to fit into the little case. My dad sits down on the floor next to me and asks me if Brian has stolen my comic books. I tell him I don't know. I say I can't remember how many were here before. My dad reaches down and curls his big hand around one of the magazines, holding it between us and asking me what it's about. I shrug. He is silent. I welcome this comfortable silence with my dad, the silence of home. Even though my life is different now, everything seems the same as we sit here. He still loves me more than anyone else in the world. Finally, he pushes himself off the floor.

"Dad?" I ask. My voice cracks.

He looks back at me.

"Do you think we could put some of this stuff away tomorrow?" I ask, waving my hand toward my kitchen appliances. "Maybe in the attic?"

He simply nods like he's not surprised by my request. The oak door scrapes across the carpet as he closes it behind him.

Attendance

My FIRST insulin reaction at school is the worst. My hands start to shake and it feels like ants are crawling on my skin. I tell myself that I can make it until lunch, but my eyes close. Mrs. Anderson acts fast, shaking my shoulder and helping me into the hall. All the kids are staring at me. The teacher's stale breath is hot on my face as she talks loudly, asking me if I'm feeling faint. Through a haze, I stare at the yellow stains on her teeth and nod. My knees are shaking and my tennis shoes squeak as we walk toward the nurse's office.

The nurse slips a piece of candy into my mouth and calls my mother who tells her to give me a piece of candy. I want to complain about the root beer flavor, but I shut up because my mom is on the line. I just want to go back to class. The other kids will be talking. The nurse places the telephone receiver in my hand and says my mother wants to talk to me.

"Don't you have any candy?" my mom asks. She sounds busy.

I tell her obviously I don't. I lift my weak arm into the air and tell her that's why I'm here. The nurse raises her eyebrows.

"You've got to take them off your dresser in the morning," my mother informs me. Then she sighs. "Don't forget tomorrow."

I tell her I won't. I just want to get off the phone and get back to my classroom. The teacher has left me behind with this woman in white.

"Okay, honey," my mom says. She tells me to cooperate with the nurse and we'll talk about it tonight. I hand the black telephone receiver back to the nurse and bite down on the candy between my teeth.

The nurse keeps me in her office for almost an hour, asking me questions about diabetes. I make up stories about how badly I was treated in the hospital. The school nurse craves drama. She wants to know the names of the nurses who worked on my floor and acts like she knows them all personally. She nods her head when I tell her they wouldn't feed me. She's pathetic. Finally, I remind her I need to get back to class. The other kids are probably talking about me. When I return to my classroom, my friend tells me the teacher explained diabetes to the fourth-grade class while I was gone. They had a half-hour discussion about insulin, injections, diabetes, and me. I blame my fourth-grade teacher when Shannon starts teasing me about being diabetic.

SHANNON follows me around during recess and makes imaginary needles with his fingers, pretending to give himself shots. He saunters up to me as I play on the jungle gym and asks me if I'm going to steal someone else's pancreas. Then he laughs and pokes himself in the arm again. My mother always says people who make fun of other people don't like themselves. His stringy black hair clings to his dirty face. The brown corduroys he wears every day are too tight and only reach to the middle of his ankles. I hate him. But my mom tells me not to say the word *hate,* so I can't tell him. He reminds me that his grandmother lost her feet to diabetes. Then he gets down on his knees, pretending not to have any lower legs, and tells me that I'm going to look like that someday. I go home and tell my mom.

My mother calls the principal who says he'll take care of the student, but Shannon continues to torment me. I dread recess every day, knowing that no matter where I go he will find me before the end of the break. With my back pressed against the chain link fence on the edge of the playground, I watch for him, hoping that he will be so engrossed in a basketball game that he'll forget about me. I've seen him tease other kids, and he'll eventually lose interest in me. I pray he finds a new person to pick on, but he doesn't.

"I've GOT this problem," I say to Denise the next Saturday afternoon. We're carrying shopping bags through the mall.

She stops in front of a store window and waits for me to continue.

"What is it?" she asks.

"Well," I begin, avoiding her eyes. "I have this kid at school teasing me."

"Teasing you about what?"

The concern in her voice silences me.

"What's she teasing you about?" Denise repeats.

"It's a boy," I reply.

"You're being teased about a boy?" She forces back a smile.

"No," I continue. "It's a boy teasing me."

"Oh. And?" she asks. I focus on a sporting goods display behind the glass. A mannequin dressed in a football jersey looks back at me. My sister's reflection looms behind me, waiting for an explanation. Juggling the shopping bags that are cutting into her wrists, she reaches up and pushes the hair away from her face. She tilts her head to see what I'm staring at. I wish now I had kept quiet.

"About diabetes," I finally reply, taking one last glance at the soccer ball before walking away. "He teases me about being diabetic. He follows me around at recess and tells me the doctor is going to cut off my feet."

Denise is silent and I can feel her anger as we approach a group of shoppers. Her movements are sharp as she darts around the crowd next to a food stand.

"You want something to drink?" she asks.

I nod and read the sign behind the counter. The cashier doesn't make change unless you buy something.

Denise pays for two pops and we sit down on a nearby bench. She tells me about a classmate in junior high who started a rumor that Denise would faint if she ate a piece of candy.

"The kids were so stupid," she says. "They believed her. Little pieces of candy kept popping up on my desk at school."

"What did you do to her?" I ask. My sister is tough and I wait for an exciting tale of bloody revenge.

"Mom called her mom," she replies.

I look over at my sister sitting next to me on the marble bench. My mother told me that when Denise was in fifth grade a student started a rumor that diabetes was contagious, and none of the kids would play with my sister. Even the parents were afraid to have her in their homes for birthday parties, scared she would pass out and they would be responsible. I always thought Denise had just beaten the other kids up.

"Oh," I reply.

Giggling teenage girls rush by us and a name is announced over the PA system. A child has been lost and they are looking for a father.

"It really sucks when people know about the disease," she continues.

I nod in agreement and sip from the blue and white straw.

"Maybe you ought to just knock him one the next time he says something to you," she suggests.

DENISE TAKES care of the problem though. She calls the school and arranges for a visiting day, an afternoon when parents can come and observe the classroom. We are studying multiplication tables when she walks into my classroom. My teacher greets her with a smile, and my sister takes an empty seat in the back of the room, scanning the students for the dark-complected boy. He squirms in his seat as she glares at him. The teacher doesn't notice.

During our lunch recess, Denise sits on the swings with me and asks what I want her to do. The wind blows her dark hair away from her round face. Sunglasses shade her eyes as she looks from me to Shannon who is playing basketball thirty feet away. I shrug and stare down at the sand. After a while, she pats my leg and tells me she'll see me next weekend. As she fumbles for her keys and heads for the car, my stomach drops.

Then she just stops. She turns around to face the kids on the court and walks straight into the middle of their game. She pulls Shannon aside by the arm. I look around for a teacher, but I know my sister doesn't care if anyone sees her. She squeezes Shannon's arm tightly and whispers something in his ear. Even though his back is to me, I know he's wiping tears from his eyes with his sleeve. He doesn't tease me again.

The bathrooms are the biggest difference between grade school and junior high. The door is marked LADIES instead of GIRLS. There are tampon machines, more mirrors, and the ceiling is higher. Hand dryers replace the rough brown paper towels I used last year. Groups of older girls gather in the corner, share lipsticks, and whisper. I get in and out of the rest room quickly. Nothing is familiar. A few of my friends are at this school, but now there are three separate lunch periods and I don't get to eat with them. I pass people I know in the hall, but there's no time to talk. Everyone rushes. And everyone is taller.

Trying to hide, I bury my head inside my locker and study the map of the building my homeroom teacher gave me. Denise said I shouldn't let anyone see it. When she was in junior high, the new kids were recognized by the yellow map. If the older kids figure out this is my first year, they'll try to sell me an elevator pass. Denise reminded me that this is a one-story building and I shouldn't fall for any of their tricks. I have to be careful, act natural. I tried to memorize the locations of my classes last week. Denise walked me through the building before school started, telling me stories of her years at Meredith Junior High. When I told her the building was too big, she said it would get smaller. She said a lot of things seem more intimidating than they really are the first time we're faced with them.

My French teacher is big-boned and graying, but her voice is soft. There's a small, circular Band-Aid stuck to her left cheek. She places her hands on her hips and tells the class to find a partner and share what school we came from, any French words we know, and why we chose French instead of Spanish. I slowly turn my head and lock eyes with the girl next to me. We choose each other, knowing that if we don't make the claim now, we might be left without a partner. There's nothing worse than being paired up by the teacher. It's like being the last one chosen for a team in soccer. I raise my eyebrows and nod to the girl. She smiles. Her teeth are a little crooked in the front and her hair is curly. She looks like a dark-haired version of Annie, the orphan, and I laugh when she tells me her name is Ann. I tell her my dad's side of the family is from Luxembourg, a small country just east of France. And I chose French because everyone else is taking Spanish. I say "everyone else" like I'm talking about my friends, but I only know that the classes were full when I tried to sign up. I don't know any French words. Neither does Ann. Mrs. Cook moves easily around the room, listening to bits and pieces of our conversations. She raises her voice above the chatter, telling us we'll be conversing with our partners in French before the year is over. Ann rolls her eyes and smiles. I like her. We agree to be partners for the rest of the year.

We pass notes in class and talk in English when Mrs. Cook is out of earshot. We laugh at the Band-Aids on Mrs. Cook's face. We joke that maybe she's a man and she cut herself shaving. Ann's mom is a nurse and says that Mrs. Cook has skin cancer. I know enough about cancer to know I shouldn't laugh, but I do anyway. The Band-Aids show up in different places on her face every week. Ann's mom tells her that Mrs. Cook is having the cancerous spots removed. The teacher styles her hair to try to hide them, combing her bangs down over her forehead and pulling a strand of gray hair across her wrinkled cheek. She can't hide the plastic strips on her nose, and when she turns to write on the board, Ann and I look at each other, point to our noses, and giggle.

The first time Ann comes to my house, we make tea. We cut slices of cheese, apples, and pears, and spread it all out on the kitchen table. Then we sit down and talk, taking turns refilling the cups. Ann's hands are small and barely reach around my mother's ceramic mug. She tells me about her religion and growing up in a Catholic home. I'm jealous, but not of the religion. My dad doesn't speak highly of the Catholic church, but I don't tell Ann that. I'm jealous because she knows more kids at school from church. She grew up with them, going to Sunday school and Communion. We talk about God and the things her parents tell her. She says she doesn't believe all of it. I like that.

She leans forward in the kitchen chair when I pull out a syringe and insulin. I told her I was diabetic, and her mom explained to her what that means, but her eyes get big when she sees the needle. She watches carefully as I draw insulin from the vial and push the metal tip against my flesh. Then she closes her eyes and turns her head. I wait for her curiosity to get the best of her, and when she looks back at my arm, expecting it to be all over, I push the needle down. She moans but keeps her eyes glued to the surface of my skin as I ease the insulin into my body. I pull the point out and hold it up for her to see. I figure she's going to ask me if the shots hurt. I expect questions about diabetes, but she says nothing. Instead she takes the syringe from between my fingers, examines it for a moment, pushes the orange cap on, and sets it on the table between us. She goes back to telling her story about Matt, the blond boy in our French class. She's not concerned with the needle.

WE'RE STUDYING the excretory system in biology class. Mr. Perschau talks about skin. It's an organ. He waves his hands in the air and explains that our skin is our greatest protector against getting hurt, and pain and pressure points detect danger.

If we touch a hot pan or step on a piece of glass, our skin is going to let us know about it before anything inside the body is too badly damaged. Mr. Perschau saunters up and down the aisles of desks, looks down over his horn-rimmed glasses at each of our books, and flips to the right page in the chapter for us. He sets his long finger on the paragraph he's referring to. Students look down at their books and his thin hand. My book is already open. I'm interested in skin.

Mr. Perschau is younger than the rest of my teachers, and I know he hasn't been here long because my older brother doesn't know him. He doesn't lose his temper when fish from the aquarium come up missing. He's the only teacher I have who doesn't write our names on the board if we do something stupid. He laughs with us when something is funny and lets the boys come in after class to watch him dissect frogs. I like him because he understands how the body works.

He passes out sewing pins and black felt markers, telling us to draw squares on the backs of our hands. Ann nudges me and points to the girl two rows in front of us. Chris Yancey is leaning over the front of her desk and softly poking the pin into the back of Mark Bancroft's head. The girl pushes Mark's black hair around with the point and then carefully buries it underneath the thick locks. She's not poking him very hard, because he doesn't turn around, but the whole class is watching now. Someone giggles and Mr. Perschau turns around. No, he informs Chris. Touch the point lightly inside the box on your *own* hand, he says. I look around the room. My classmates push the pins into the black boxes. They glance up at Mr. Perschau for approval, unsure of what exactly this experiment is demonstrating. I understand perfectly. I touch the metal tip to my skin. Some places I feel pain and some places I don't.

I DROP MY backpack on the bathroom floor and sit on the edge of the bathtub. Folding my leg to my chest, I pull the orange cap off a syringe with my teeth. I steady my arm with the back of my knee and touch the metal to my skin. I push the point around the surface of the skin until I find a spot where I can't feel the prick. When I come to a place where the needle is met with no feeling, I bury it beneath the surface of my skin. I don't rotate the injection site like I'm supposed to, and I never use alcohol to clean the area. I know the standard procedure for an injection, but my way is faster. And now it's virtually painless. I know the doctors and nurses wouldn't approve of my method. They would tell me I'm contaminating the needle, but I don't follow their rules anymore.

My skin is paying for it. I give my shots in my left arm every day. The tissue over my triceps has hardened. It looks like an overdeveloped muscle. Too many needles pushed into the same area for too long result in a lump of scar tissue. If I hold my arm straight out and twist it up so the triceps face the ceiling, an unnatural bump sticks out.

When I first was diagnosed with diabetes, the nurses stressed the importance of rotation, telling me if I didn't frequently change the location of the injection, the tissue would become hard. They gave me strips of paper with holes cut out about every inch. They told me to set the paper on my legs, upper arm, or abdomen and insert the needle into a different circle every time. But the back of my left arm is the most comfortable spot. I can fold my left leg up against my chest, set the back of my upper arm on my knee, and pop the needle in and out with my right hand. It's the easiest place, and there aren't any nurses around to tell me I'm doing it wrong. Most of the time they don't know what they're talking about anyway. They don't live with the disease.

Only my sister and I do. When I show Denise what I learned in biology, she runs her finger over her eyebrow and tells me I'm clever. I want her to try it out with her needles too. She says she will, but I know she won't. She has her own routine. And her skin pays for it too. Denise has been giving her shots in the same area on her thigh all her life. She says the big lump doesn't matter anymore. Too many years have passed. The skin just below where the leg and hip meet is atrophied. A mound of scar tissue protrudes, but she won't put the needle anywhere else. My mom says that's where the old, dull hypodermic syringes were inserted when Denise was little. No one taught them the rotation method in the 1960s, and twenty-five years later, Denise won't push the needle down anywhere else in her body.

NEXT TO my name on every school attendance sheet, the clinical term "diabetes mellitus" is written. The teachers try to hide the side note from my view, but I know it's there. My teachers never ask me any questions when I say I'm not feeling well. If I tell them I didn't get my homework done because I was sick, they give me a sympathetic nod and credit for the unfinished assignment. If I rub my temple like my head hurts, they ask me if I want to go see the school nurse. Sometimes it's embarrassing, but usually I take them up on the offer. The old woman in the small office listens to my heart and lets me lie on the cot and close my eyes. It's better than sitting in the classroom.

The one teacher who doesn't accept my excuses is my government teacher. Mr. Drummond stands about six five and has a mass of gray, curly hair and thick glasses over his wild eyes. Everyone fears his temper. He thinks we should know the Constitution by heart. He rambles on about our rights to free speech and how we might not realize the importance of it now, but it would matter to us if it was taken away. Mr. Drummond targets students with questions like, "What if I told you you couldn't put a Nativity scene in your yard during Christmas?" or, "What if you had to go to jail for burning a flag?" The burning-the-flag idea gets some of the students' attention. A few kids raise their hands and tell stories of their grandfathers and fathers fighting for our country. The boy in the back row with a baseball cap sitting crooked on his head says he'd beat up anyone who burned the flag around him. Mr. Drummond shakes his head and interrupts the kid, changing the discussion to the issues of symbolism and freedom of expression. Mr. Drummond calls me "Dominick" and tells me to pay attention, stop passing notes to my friends, sit up straight at my desk. No one is dumb enough to let themselves fall asleep in his class.

My friend Kelly closed her eyes in his class once. He was explaining how a bill becomes a law, and complaining about the governor of Iowa. He has this way of turning lectures about governmental procedures into commentaries on our elected officials. My sister warned me that he uses his desk as a soapbox. He spotted Kelly sleeping, and his eyes kept darting back to her every few seconds as he talked to the rest of the class. We all knew he was watching her, but the prospect of some excitement kept us from waking her up. Mr. Drummond intentionally allowed her to descend deeper and deeper into sleep. Finally, he picked up his leather-bound copy of *American Government and the Constitution* and walked toward her desk, still speaking to the rest of the class as if nothing was different. He raised the book over his head and slammed it down on Kelly's wooden desk, missing her skull by an inch. She shot straight up and was met with his eyes. Then he flashed a satisfied smile, nodded, and continued his lecture.

I know I have to keep my eyes wide open and straight ahead during his class, but as he reads the class an article about a candidate for governor, my eyelids fall. His monotone voice drones in the background of my dream. The next thing I know he's tapping lightly on my shoulder, calling me by my first name. I open my eyes and everyone is staring at me. A look of worry spreads across Mr. Drummond's usually scary face. I look into his eyes. Up close I see dried mucus and concern. No book slamming down on my desk. No asking me to stand up in the back of the room for the rest of the hour. No extra assignment to complete for the next day. Mr. Drummond leans down and whispers in my ear, "Do you need some sugar?" I shake my head, sit straight up, and stare at the chalkboard.

A few of the girls in class make a smacking noise with their lips. I look at Ann. She's turned around in her seat, eyes nar-rowed, studying me. I narrow my eyes back at her and she smiles. She knows I'm just tired. It's not an insulin reaction, but I want Mr. Drummond to think it is, so I reach into my pocket and pull a peppermint pinwheel out. I make sure he's looking at me as I place the candy on my tongue. Maybe I'm taking advantage of my illness, but I know the other kids would do the same thing. I crinkle the plastic wrapper between my fingers.

Rejecting the Needle

AIDS CHANGES my relationship with the needle. The insulin injector has become an HIV transmitter. My friends still look at the needle with wonder, but they fear the metal tip more than when we were in grade school. We learn all about AIDS in home economics. The elderly teacher looks nervous when she tells us the disease doesn't belong to gay men, it belongs to kids our age. The topic of sex usually makes us giggle, but no one laughs when the teacher tells us HIV is transmitted through semen. Anal sex. Oral sex. Even the boys in the back of the room shift in their seats and look down at their hands. Don't have sex without a condom. Don't share needles.

No one is too concerned about the needles part. Using intravenous drugs doesn't even occur to us. Sex, on the other hand, makes our ears perk up. We're old enough now to be having sex. Or at least the school must think so or they wouldn't be telling us about AIDS. I'm familiar with the fleeting fear this kind of talk arouses. We will each walk out of here and think it will never happen to us. We're young and just starting our lives. Bad things happen to other people. If you don't truly fear it, it can't happen to you.

The teacher looks relieved as she wheels a metal cart to the front of the classroom. A television is stacked on top of a VCR. A video about AIDS. A man in a black suit narrates, holds up condom packages, tells us what not to do. Then an emaciated young man holding a syringe appears on the screen. The plastic needle looks just like one of mine. The man is dying. Propped in a chair and rolling the syringe between his fingers, he tells the camera that he's eighteen years old. He says he never thought this would happen to him. He talks about his girlfriend and the college he'll never attend. He wishes he had the chance to live his life over, live it differently. My eyes are fixed on the man's sunken chest, and I can't pull my gaze away from the screen to see the expression on my classmates' faces. But I know they associate the needle with death now.

I'm careless with my syringes. On the floor of my locker, at the bottom of my backpack, under my bed at home, a needle can be found. I seem to leave a trail of them wherever I go. A few years ago, it wasn't a big deal, but now people fear them. Ann tells me to break the metal tips off and put them in the garbage can. She says I have to start disposing of them properly.

My mom tells me this too. I'm supposed to put the syringes in a Planters Peanut jar that sits on the bathroom vanity. No more needles in the bathroom trash can. My dad tapes a little circle of white paper to the jar above the little peanut man's head. It says, "Bring me your needles." I smile when I look at it, but I always drop my syringes in the trash can. I know the next time my mom walks into the bathroom she's going to bend down, shake her head in disgust, and pull them out. She places the syringes in the peanut jar and then seals the airtight lid. There's no escape for them. I tell my mom she's paranoid. She says she read a story about a garbageman suing a diabetic when he got pricked with one of her needles while collecting garbage. He contracted hepatitis or something. When I ask where she read the story, she replies she can't remember. I tell her she dreamed it up. I'm not going to gather up all my needles and seal them in a glass jar.

———

I place the glucometer on the bathroom vanity and rub my fingers together, stimulating the circulation in my hands. The urine tests for detecting sugar used to be easier, but they weren't as accurate as this machine. Now I use a drop of blood to give me an exact reading. I puncture the end of my pinkie with the jagged, metal lancet and wipe my bloody finger on the end of a test strip. The machine beeps and I push the strip into the slot. Forty-five seconds. The digital numbers count it down for me. I gaze into the mirror.

There are three pimples on my forehead that my bangs don't cover. I pull the hair down to my eyebrows, but it parts in the middle and exposes the red blotches. My mom says they never go away because I pick at them, but I pick at them to make them go away. When Denise was in high school, she used to fill her syringes with peroxide and push the needles under her pimples. She stood in front of the bathroom mirror, twisted the white cap off the bottle of peroxide, and poured the liquid into it. Then she filled the syringe up and carefully poked it into the skin on her face. My mom used to stand in the doorway and shake her head, telling my sister the needle would scar her face. It didn't. The pimple bubbled and dried out by the next day.

The machine beeps and the digital screen reads "high." One hundred is average, and this machine only reads to 400. I'm off the charts, but I'm not surprised. I haven't given a shot for four days. I'm trying to lose weight, and I figure giving up insulin is the easiest way. I still eat, but my body can't use the food. I push the Off button on the machine and zip the vinyl case around it. I pull a syringe from a package in the closet, take off the plastic wrapper, and drop it in the trash can. It lands on top of crumpled tissues. My mother won't get suspicious.

My parents will send me to the hospital or punish me if they find out I'm not giving my shots. As far as I know, Denise never rejected the needle when she was my age. I thought this one up on my own. If my sister finds out, she'll lecture me. She's in graduate school now and throws big parties on the weekends, staying up late and drinking with her friends. But she always gives her shots. She smokes and drinks and doesn't exercise, but she always pushes the needle into her leg. The shots keep her grounded.

I spend more time with Denise now that I'm a teenager. She helps me write papers for school and talks to me about boys and sex. My mother lets me sleep over at her house, and I stay with her on the weekends when my parents leave town. Brian has started his first year of college, and my parents won't let me stay alone overnight yet. They tell me maybe next year. My mother says she trusts me but not some of my friends. She tells me I have to be careful not to let the rest of the group influence me too much. I argue with her that peer pressure is a phrase coined by adults so they don't have to blame their kids for doing stupid things. She replies that maybe I have a point, but she's still not going to leave me in the house by myself for a weekend.

I know my parents trust me. They don't hassle me about studying like Ann's parents do her. All my dad says is that I'll want to get into college in a few years and I'll be sorry if I don't keep my grades up now. I don't think about the future much. College seems like a lifetime away, and the world of adults isn't too appealing. Ann and I think about moving to Minneapolis or Paris and working in a boutique. That sounds more exciting than college. When I mention the idea to my dad, he suggests we wait until after we get degrees in business or marketing. He doesn't really worry about me though. He says I'm more responsible than Brian and Denise were at my age.

My dad asks me questions about my boyfriend though. Jeff is a year older than me and has a car. Even though my dad likes him, I don't think he trusts him. Denise says it's a "father thing." My dad acted the same way with Denise when she started dating. My sister tells me he'll grow out of it. He just loves me too much. Denise says having a boyfriend reminds my dad that someday I'll have a husband. It's hard for parents to let their kids go.

My parents would be more upset about me not giving shots than if I brought a D home in algebra. But I need to lose weight—Jeff is looking at skinnier girls. My 110-pound body is too fat compared to the girl I saw Jeff talking to last week. He was playing basketball outside the school with his friends, and when I showed up, the girl walked away. She was tall and blond and very thin. Her shorts were too tight, and I would have made fun of them if Ann had been with me. I was alone. When I asked Jeff who she was, he shrugged and replied that he didn't know her name. He looked nervous though, and his eyes darted in her direction as she walked away. I crossed my arms in front of my chest and narrowed my eyes at him. He was about to come up with some explanation when one of his friends threw the ball and smacked Jeff in the bare shoulder. He turned his back on me and dribbled across the concrete, his shorts falling down to his hipbones. I watched the girl walking away. I'm not going to dye my hair blond, but I am going to lose five pounds. Maybe ten. I have an advantage.

Diabetes has its benefits. I can force my body to feed on itself if I don't give it any insulin. I risk acidosis, but I don't really understand exactly what that is anyway. I remember the little white pills and the way my parents hoped they wouldn't change color, but they never explained what was happening to my body if the pill turned purple. High blood sugars for long periods of time can cause damage to my body, but I'm young. My sister is still healthy, and she's had diabetes a lot longer than I have.

———————

I open my eyes and look down at myself. An IV drips clear fluid into my arm, and an electronic machine next to the bed records my heart rate. A blood pressure cup tightens around my biceps every few minutes. The neckline of my hospital gown is frayed; hard, crisp sheets rub against my bare feet. A pale man holding a clipboard stares down at me.

"What happened?" he asks. "Did you stop giving your shots?"

Looking around the room for my parents, I shrug innocently. Every muscle in my body aches and my feet are cold. A sour-tasting film coats the inside of my mouth. Staring at the stethoscope dangling around his neck, I avoid looking up at his face. The red stripes on his tie clash with the yellow button-down shirt beneath the familiar doctor's coat. His eyes burn through the top of my head.

"How did I get here?" I ask. "Where are my parents?"

"You didn't wake up this morning," he informs me. "When your mom tried to get you up for school, you wouldn't respond."

I wait for a more thorough explanation, but he just stares at me.

"Your blood sugar was over five hundred," he states, pointing his finger at the chart. "There was alcohol in your bloodstream. You tell me how you got here."

I close my heavy eyes, feigning fatigue, waiting for him to leave.

"Have you been giving any insulin at all?" he asks.

"Of course I have," I lie.

He turns his back to me. I watch as he shakes his head the way doctors do, slowly from side to side. He is young and his blond hair is cut short. The back of his neck is cleanly shaven.

"You've been diabetic almost five years now?" he asks, facing me again.

"I suppose that's what the chart says," I reply.

"Do you understand what your disease is?" he asks. "Do you know how important it is to keep your blood sugar stable?"

I roll my eyes.

"At the rate you're going, you'll be lucky to live another five," he states. "I'm going to be straight with you. Whatever it is you're doing, or not doing, you're going to end up sorry. Young diabetics come in here every day with problems. They're going blind and their kidneys are failing because they aren't taking care of themselves." He pauses. "You are a perfect candidate for complications."

I wonder where my parents are. Thinking back to the night before, I remember coming home from Ann's house. Her parents were out for dinner and a bunch of kids from school were there. We were watching movies and everyone was drinking. Jeff brought beer and a bottle of vodka. About ten o'clock, I started feeling sick and Jeff drove me home. My mother was curled up in a chair watching the news when I walked into the house. My dad glanced from his book over the top of his glasses at me. He asked me how my night had been. Having told them I was going to Ann's to study, I replied that I got a lot of work done. I threw my backpack down in the corner of the living room and got ready for bed. I was exhausted and fell asleep with the radio on.

"You know you could have died this morning?" he asks. "Why don't you tell me what you've been doing."

I want to tell him that I'm tired of it all. The shots, the tests, the doctors' appointments. My friends eat lunch at donut shops without worrying about their blood sugars. I just want to do the things that they're doing, but this man standing over me won't understand. When Ann asks me questions about my diabetes or expresses concern over whether or not I'm eating right, I tell her it is no big deal. I'm sick of the tedious routine of being a diabetic, sick of following it, sick of talking about it. I keep my mouth closed and stare at the wall.

"Were you trying to lose weight?" he asks.

I look up at him.

"Do I look like I need to lose weight?" I ask.

"No," he replies. "I'm just trying to figure out how your blood sugars got so high. People your age stop giving their shots for crazy reasons."

He talks just like an adult and just like a doctor. I want to tell him he doesn't know anything, but my mother walks in. She sits on the edge of the hospital bed and pats my leg, telling me everything will be okay. Tests reported that my kidneys haven't been damaged and my blood sugar is finally stable. They've been slowly dripping insulin into my IV the last few hours. Her eyes are full of tears and questions she doesn't ask.

My father hovers in the doorway talking with the doctor. With his hand resting against his cheek, he nods in agreement with whatever the man is saying. The jacket of his favorite gray suit hangs over his arm and the back of his dress shirt is untucked. He has rushed from his office to the hospital, and tension is cramping the muscles in his shoulders. The worried expression on his face turns to disappointment as the doctor talks.

The room closes in around me and the uniform beeping of the machines lulls my eyes closed. A nurse gently cradles my arm, touching the needle of the IV lightly. Her soft hands are warm and she whispers something to my mother. I'm suddenly comfortable in this hard bed with the sheets tucked too tightly around my legs. Carts are wheeled by and telephones ring in the distance.

The nurses let me rest the first day, checking in on me every few hours and ordering blood work. I push the words of the blond doctor to the back of my mind and think about the last week. It has been eight days since I've given a shot. Maybe nine, I can't remember. Each morning when I opened the drawer in the bathroom to pull out my toothbrush, two half-empty bottles of insulin looked back at me. I don't know why I didn't just draw the insulin into the syringe, but it got easier to ignore the glass bottles with each day. The longer I went without giving a shot, the more futile it had seemed to start giving them again. Now my body has failed me.

The doctors keep me in the hospital three days, regulating my blood sugar and reminding me how to count food exchanges and inject the correct dosage of insulin. They tell me stories about faceless diabetic teenagers who have been through their intensive care unit. I remain motionless on the bed as they recount the tales of a thirteen-year-old girl who is losing her vision and a seventeen-year-old who died from a heart attack. They try to frighten me into taking care of myself, but I'm familiar with their tactics.

Ann comes to visit me the second day. She walks into my room with a balloon tied around her wrist, takes one look at me propped up in bed, and starts to cry. Her mother probably told her I've done a bad thing. Ann's mom always tells her about advances made in diabetes, and Ann informs me of the medical breakthroughs. When the insulin pump was developed, she brought an article to school with a picture attached. She said she thought it was a good idea to keep my blood sugar stable. I looked down at the picture and back at her concerned face. I told her I wouldn't carry a box around on the side of my body. The needle works just fine. But I rebelled against the needle, and Ann's angry with me for not taking care of myself. Pulling the tan padded chair from the corner, she sits close to my bed and listens as I confess what I've done. She closes her eyes and shakes her head, telling me I have been stupid. I wish she didn't know so much.

Jeff looks lost when he enters my hospital room. He squints and blinks twice before he fully realizes it's me curled up in the bed. Then he walks slowly toward me, like he's afraid to get too close.

"Hi there," he says.

I force a smile.

"What happened?" he asks.

"Nothing really. I just got sick and they're making a big deal out of it."

He looks down at the IV in my arm and the heart monitor attached to my chest.

"Well, I guess it must be a pretty big deal if they're keeping you here," he replies. "Is it the diabetes?"

The diabetes.

"No," I lie, knowing he only believes me because he wants to. "I'll be out of here tomorrow."

I don't tell him anything else. The less he understands about the illness, the less he'll question me about it. The first three months we dated, he didn't even know I was diabetic. Finally, he spotted a needle in the bottom of my purse and asked me what it was for. I nonchalantly responded that I was diabetic and quickly changed the topic. I don't want him to think about it. My relationship with him is not the same as my relationship with Ann. Jeff seems more conditional. Ann says my reasons for not telling him are subconscious—that I believe he won't want to be with me because I'm not the healthiest mate to bear his children. It's not that; I just don't want him to know. He'll start looking at me the way Ann does if I choose regular Coke instead of diet Coke at a restaurant. I get annoyed when people ask me if I remembered to give my shot or whether or not I should be eating a Snickers candy bar. What do they think I'm going to do? Say no I shouldn't and throw the candy bar in the garbage can?

Jeff sits on the edge of my hospital bed and we talk about our friends. He tells me about a student who drove his car across the school lawn yesterday. The homecoming dance is the next weekend and kids are having big parties. With my back pressed against the crisp pillowcase, I reassure Jeff that I will be back for all the activities. Relief spreads across his face. The relief of ignorance.

WHEN I GET home, my parents watch me more closely. I don't get in trouble for what I did or have to give my shots in front of them, but I can feel them watching me. My mom pulls the glucometer from the back of the bathroom cupboard and sets it on the shelf every morning. I test my blood sugar before school. The words of the doctor scared me, but I never admit that to anyone. I tell Ann I'm going to take better care of myself because I want to, not because I'm worried about the future. She says, "Whatever." She doesn't care what reason I come up with to do it. She worries enough for the both of us.

Old Enough

THE NURSE pulls the needle from a vein in my inner arm and applies pressure to the spot with a cotton ball. Her eyes tell me to hold it in place as she bends my arm. With gloved hands, she picks up the vial of blood and turns away from me without a word. The heavy door clicks closed behind her, and my eyes scan the familiar office. The same art hangs on the wall, Dr. Manning's cracked brown stool stands in the corner, and the glass jars filled with cotton balls are untouched. I know this place.

Each year before school starts, my mother takes me to Dr. Manning's small office for a physical and blood work, but as I sit waiting for him today, I'm alone. My mother doesn't know about this appointment. I am pregnant. The family planning clinic in Des Moines won't perform an abortion on me without consent from my primary physician. They don't want to be responsible for individuals with health complications. The woman at the clinic told me diabetics need special permission to obtain an abortion there. She said I was more prone to infections, might have problems maintaining normal blood-sugar levels, and could need more aftercare than a nondiabetic woman after an abortion.

I am seventeen years old. Almost eighteen. Old enough to

have a baby, I think, and I know the risks. Not just to my education and future but to my health. I've heard the horror stories of diabetic mothers. My blood sugars haven't been as closely controlled as they need to be for a pregnancy, and this could put both me and the fetus in jeopardy.

Dr. Manning knocks once and enters. He stands less than five nine, not much taller than me, and his hair has gotten longer since the last time I saw him. He looks ten years younger than he is. He reminds me of a hippie disguised in a white coat, and his plaid tennis shoes catch my eye. Even though he's easy-going, the sight of him always makes me nervous. I have known him most of my life, but he's still the potential bearer of bad news. I'm never sure how I'll feel at the end of our visit, and my blood pressure is always high in this office. He tells me it is the "white coat syndrome," but he doesn't know why I get it. He says I should feel at home here, surrounded by the watercolor series hanging on the wall. He painted the pictures himself.

"Hey, kiddo," he says, winking at me and setting my chart down on the counter.

I force a smile.

"What brings you here? Looks like your Pap smear results came back fine and your blood sugars were up last time, but I'm not going to lecture you about that again." He flips through the pages of my thick folder and glances up at me.

"I'm pregnant."

I just say it. Like I'm reciting lines from a movie. I've been taking birth control pills for over a year, swallowing one little pink tablet every morning when I give a shot. I don't know how this happened; I never miss a dose. Dr. Manning doesn't ask. My heart beats hard against my chest. I can't look him in the eye, so I stare at the beige carpet. Words tumble from my lips.

"They told me at the clinic that I had to have your okay to get an abortion. You know. They're scared of the complications associated with diabetes or something. I was there and ready to go through with it, but when they did a blood sugar it came back high. Then they got mad that I hadn't told them I was diabetic to begin with. Like I was lying on purpose or trying to pull one over. I didn't know it was a big deal."

Dr. Manning takes a deep breath and runs his hand over the back of his neck before acknowledging what I've said. I shift my gaze to the wall, knowing the compassion in his brown eyes will bring tears to my own.

I told myself I wouldn't cry. Said I'd be strong through this whole thing. I'm a kid, too young to have a baby. I blink my eyes quickly. It's the stress, I reassure myself. It's the stress and I'm tired and I'm worried and that's why my eyes are filling up with tears. I look down at my shoes. They look like blurry, brown puddles.

"They've got to be careful to protect both you and the agency," he begins. "How far along did they say you were?"

"Almost ten weeks, so they let me go ahead and schedule for next Wednesday. But they said I had to have consent from you or they wouldn't perform the procedure, and I've already been throwing up in the morning."

But it's more than just normal morning sickness that is making me ill. Throwing up every time I eat results in insulin reactions, and I almost passed out twice during my journalism class. My sweaty skin is sticking to the sheets on my bed when I wake up in the morning. I feel strange. Weak. Infected. Like my body is rejecting what's happening to it, is angry with me.

Dr. Manning pulls his rusty stool from the corner and slides up next to me. With his face close to mine, I am forced to look into his eyes.

"Are you sure an abortion is what you want to do? You're a senior now, right?" he asks.

I nod.

"How have your blood sugars been?"

I lie that I think they're doing okay. He just frowns at me, as if he knows I'm not checking them like I should be or am just not telling him the truth.

"And you've thought about this a lot?" he asks, the words sounding more like a statement than a question.

I nod again.

He pauses, exhaling loudly before he continues.

"Not everyone has to have children, Andie. Not every woman should have them. It's not a rule that because you're female you have to bear a child," he says, never taking his eyes from mine. "So many young people now getting pregnant. Rushing into having babies." He shakes his head and flips through my file. His eyes are met with pages and pages of blood test results and examination records.

"I just hope you're testing your blood sugars. We don't want you to end up in the hospital again," he says.

"I know," I say under my breath.

"Same boyfriend?" he asks.

"Yes." I talked to Dr. Manning about Jeff last year when I started taking the pill.

"Does he know?"

"No," I reply.

Jeff is 300 miles away at college. I haven't talked to him in over a week and know if I tell him he'll want to get married. He'd say it is the right thing to do. He has always said he will marry me if I ever get pregnant, assuming that eases some fear in me.

"I don't want to marry him," I continue. "I don't want to get married."

Dr. Manning takes my elbow in his hand. He lightly touches my fingers that have been holding the cotton ball on my arm in place. I realize I've been putting so much pressure on it, my whole arm aches. He slowly pulls the cotton ball off and looks at the mark the needle has left on my inner arm. Pushing down the pedal on the garbage can with his plaid shoe, he drops the stained cotton inside. A small drop of blood forms on my skin. Reaching up and pulling a clean cotton ball from the glass jar, he secures it to my arm with a Band-Aid.

"I'm just too young," I say. "I know I want to do other things. Things that don't include being married or babies."

"Have you told your mom and dad?"

"No," I say. "Not yet."

He doesn't respond and the silence in the room is suddenly awkward. Through the door I hear a nurse giving instructions to another patient. Step on the scale and stand up straight, she says. Dr. Manning turns his head toward the sound of her voice and pauses before looking back at me.

"Okay, kiddo. Well, you know that this is ultimately your decision and I'll support you in whatever you want to do. I don't want you to think you can't have children because you're diabetic though. If you're going to undergo an abortion it should be because you—your mind, not just your body—don't want to have a child. He sets his hand gently on the top of my head. "And there's adoption to think about. You have to consider all your options. The main thing I'm concerned about is what you've been doing for the last few months. If you've been running high blood sugars, that complicates things in carrying a child to term. You know that."

I know.

"But," he continues, exhaling loudly again, "I'll write you a consent and you can take the next week or so to think about it. You want to decide before you get to the twelve-week mark though."

Dr. Manning goes on to explain the risks of diabetic pregnancies, particularly to the fetus in the first three months. A closely regulated blood sugar is crucial during this time to prevent possible birth defects. Even if a diabetic mother is extremely careful throughout the pregnancy, complications may ensue. By having a baby, I could risk my own health and longevity more than anything. Blindness and kidney failure are sometimes the results of a diabetic woman's giving birth to a child. Pregnancy can put a strain on the circulatory system as well as all the major organs in the body. He says that if I decide to have the child, he will refer me to an OB/GYN who specializes in diabetic pregnancies, but he looks at me like he knows the referral won't be necessary. The expression on my face reflects that my mind is made up.

I tell Dr. Manning that I know a diabetic woman who has two children and is fine. He explains the difference to me. That I am different. Unplanned pregnancies for diabetics can be catastrophic. I'm reminded of the movie *Steel Magnolias*. Julia Roberts plays a diabetic who suffers kidney failure and eventually dies after the birth of her son. She undergoes kidney dialysis and her inner arms resemble railroad tracks from the treatments. I envision myself holding my child, and my arms belong to Julia Roberts. I think about touching the cheek of a baby I can't see because I've gone blind, of my child attending my funeral before she is able to understand what a funeral is. The image of my father standing in front of my casket fills my head. And I contemplate the value of my own life, wondering how much I'll ever be willing to sacrifice to have a baby.

My sister is almost thirty and doesn't have any children. She never talks about kids, avoids even looking at them when we're in public. About a year ago, we were shopping and I asked her if she wanted a baby. She didn't answer my question and continued to flip through the rack of jeans and hum a song like she hadn't heard me. I believed that if she had a baby, maybe I'd eventually have one too. But she hasn't. She's too scared.

Not everyone should have children. Those words echo in my head as I push open the outer doors of Dr. Manning's office. Instead of getting in my car and heading back to class, I walk across the parking lot to an empty football field. The sky is rumbling and rain threatens to fall at any moment. I spread my body out on the cool grass and watch the clouds darken above me. Running my hands over my stomach, I whisper to the entity in my belly. Rain begins to fall and I blink to clear my vision. The drops come larger and faster. My hair soaks up raindrops, and the long brown strands spread out onto the earth around me. The rain cleanses me.

My clothes are covered with mud, and grass sticks to the back of my jacket when I sit up. Holding my leather backpack close to my chest, I listen to the sounds of cars whizzing by on the freeway. The grass around the football bleachers is starting to turn brown. The Iowa winter will soon return.

In the middle of this football field, with rain dripping from my eyelashes, I could be any seventeen-year-old girl skipping school. Isolation envelops me. Reaching my hand across my body, I touch the cotton ball secured to my inner arm. The wet fibers collapse under my fingers. I tuck my nail beneath the sticky Band-Aid and slowly peel the tape away. A single spot of dried blood has formed a tiny circle on the cotton ball, and my skin is bruised. I wrap my hand around the bandage and crush it. Drops fall from the white fibers onto the ground, mixing with the rain. I slip the cotton into my pocket and pick up my backpack. My tennis shoes squeak as I walk back in the direction of my car.

DENISE ISN'T shocked. She acts as though she had almost expected something like this and tries to get me to talk about my decision as she drives me to the clinic a week later. Maneuvering her red Honda through morning rush-hour traffic, she reaches over and turns the volume on the stereo down.

"How are you doing?" she asks.

I shrug and stare through the tinted glass of the window. The smoke from our cigarettes fills the car.

Denise doesn't say anything to me about smoking anymore. I stole my first cigarette from her when I was fourteen, and she made me throw it in the toilet when she caught me. I watched as the dirty butt floated around in the porcelain bowl. Denise peered over my shoulder and, with her mouth less than an inch from my ear, told me never to do it again. She sounded like my mother and I resented her. I turned around and stared at the cigarette burning between her fingers, but she reminded me that I wasn't as old as she was. Today it seems like I am. She doesn't lecture me now.

"It'll be over with in a few hours," she says. The words are meant to reassure me, but her tone sounds almost argumentative.

"I just can't believe this has all happened," I say. "I can't believe I'm doing this." I pause to light another cigarette. "God, Jeff would really be pissed."

"Yeah, well . . ." Denise's voice trails off.

My sister doesn't like Jeff. She says he doesn't care about me, doesn't understand anything about diabetes, and doesn't even try. I have tried to explain to her that it is me, not him, who never talks about it. He doesn't know anything because I haven't told him. But my sister won't accept excuses like that, replying that if people really care, they ask.

I watch the muscles in her thin neck strain as she pushes her head forward and looks into traffic. She shifts gears and accelerates through a yellow stoplight. Her seat belt isn't fastened and a burning cigarette dangles from her lips. My appointment is at eight A.M., and neither of us has taken a shower. Denise's hair is pulled back in a ponytail and her eyebrows are rumpled. She slips the Honda into neutral, slows for a red light, and looks over at me. Her eyes are studying every inch of my face.

"Who did you tell about this?" she asks.

"Ann," I reply. "And you."

"Did the nurse explain what they're going to do this morning?"

"Ann filled me in," I say.

A knot forms in my stomach as I remember the words of my friend. When I get there, I will go to the bathroom before they take me to an examination room. A doctor will feel my uterus to determine the size and position of the fetus. With local anesthesia and my legs in stirrups, they will wash me out with antiseptic. Then pressure and pain as they empty out my uterus with the aspirator. The sucking noise of the vacuum will be the worst part.

"They use a vacuum," I inform Denise.

She keeps her eyes on the road and nods.

The nurse at the clinic told me abortions are safer now. Before vacuums were used, women underwent a procedure known as dilation and curettage. Their cervixes were opened far enough to pass an instrument through and scrape out the contents of the uterus. Sometimes the uterine walls were punctured or the cervix was torn. She told me some of the women bled to death, but now, rather than scraping out the fetus, the contents are sucked through a strawlike tube. The nurse told me not to worry, and when the doctor is done my uterus will contract to its normal size. I will be my old self.

"The procedure is only supposed to take a few minutes," I continue. "I'll be able to go back to school tomorrow."

"Maybe. We'll see how you feel."

My sister called the school early this morning and told the secretary I wouldn't be in class. When I told Denise the school would never miss me, she replied that we didn't want to take any chances. She was right. I didn't want them to call my mother at work.

"It seems like everyone I know has had an abortion," I say. "Was it like that when you were in school?"

"No," she replies flatly. "It wasn't."

"But wouldn't you go through with this if you were me?" I ask.

"I guess," she sighs. "It just wasn't the same when I was in school."

I think back to my sister as a high school student. I remember her clothes in the midseventies and the way her long hair parted in the middle and hung straight down the sides of her face. She had a boyfriend with a loud car, but I can't remember his name now. He honked when he picked her up and never came inside to talk to me or my parents. My dad didn't like him, and he complained when my sister raced out of the house without saying good-bye. I remember her coming home drunk on the weekends and getting in fights with my mother. I wonder how her years in high school could have been different from mine.

Denise seems disappointed in me. Her arms are tense and her back is pushed tight against the seat of her car. She's sitting up too straight. It's like there's something she wants to say, but she's holding back. Her left leg shakes impatiently, even though traffic is moving along smoothly. I recognize this nervous habit. She's trying to be supportive, be my friend. But she can't forget that I'm still her little sister.

There's a part of me that wants her to tell me what to do. It was easier when I was younger and she gave me input on the decisions I had to make. I could rely on Denise to help me because she had been through it all. She told me how to deal with problems. But as I get older, our relationship is changing. She doesn't offer her advice as quickly anymore. She knows she has to let me grow up my own way.

We drive in uncomfortable silence. She turns the familiar corner to the clinic, and I look around for people who might know me or protesters carrying signs. They often surround the clinic, chanting Bible verses and calling the doctors and nurses inside the clinic murderers. Some days protesters lie down in the driveway here, refusing to move for the traffic until the police finally come and arrest them. My mother calls them fanatics and shakes her head at the protesters on television.

No one is here today. The parking lot is almost empty. Denise chooses a parking spot close to the door and looks over at me. Her gaze is eerily distant. She reaches for her bag in the backseat, and I know it's time. A thick hardcover book falls out, and she closes her hand too tightly around it and returns it to the black bag. Unfastening my seat belt, I lean forward and look through the windshield at the brick building. It's two stories high and the windows are all tinted black. My hands shake as I reach down onto the floor for my own purse. When I try to open the car door, the wind pushes the heavy metal back at me. Dead leaves dance against the cement curb.

Roommates

Every Sunday night at eight o'clock the phone in my dorm room rings. Both of my parents are on the line. I envision them sitting at opposite ends of the house, cradling the telephone receivers. My mom in the kitchen and my dad in his basement office. My mother asks me how I'm doing, and I remind her it's only been a week since I've spoken to her. She replies a lot can happen in a week. I agree but report that nothing has. My dad asks if they can drive up and take me to dinner on Wednesday. I tell him I have a class that night. He always forgets. Then I talk about my classes, my roommate, the food. I tell them I'm studying a lot and meeting new people. Before I hang up, they tell me they love me. I tell them I love them too, remind them I'm less than an hour from home—only forty miles away—and reassure them that they don't have to worry about me.

I worry about them. My brother is married and living in Wisconsin, and Denise rarely visits them. Sometimes, at night, I wonder what they're doing without me in the house. My roommate, Angie, tells me I'm being egocentric and that my parents are finally having sex after thirty years of living with kids. Maybe they're having the time of their lives and the Sunday night call is made out of obligation. But I can tell by the tone of my father's voice on the other end of the line that he misses me.

I miss him too. Miss home. Ann chose a university farther

north, and we exchange an occasional letter or phone call. I go out with my new friends on the weekends, learn to like beer, and master flirtation with older boys. The girls on my floor are separated into two groups, sorority and antisorority. The ones I hang out with say the Greek system is for conformists. Angie is an open lesbian, which makes for frequent propositions from the boys on the fourth floor. When they approach me and ask me if they can watch my roommate have sex with her girlfriend, I roll my eyes and tell them to grow up. When I raise my middle finger to them and turn away, I know I'm changing. The things I used to find funny now make me angry.

One afternoon Angie comes home from class, throws her backpack on the floor, and sits down on our couch. Immediately, she screams, "Shit," and jumps back up. My heart sinks when I see the syringe sticking out of the back of her thigh. She yanks it out of her leg and throws it on the floor. She runs her thick fingers through her short blond hair and calls me a careless bitch. Then she says she's sorry.

I'm not sure how to react. I have a bad habit of pulling the syringe from my arm and sticking it into furniture. I shake my head, tell her I'm sorry, pick up the needle, and start looking around for the orange cap. I can't find it. I dig between the cushions of the couch, searching, as she stands above me and rubs the back of her leg. I must look pathetic, because she tells me not to worry about it. She gives me her famous "We'll laugh about it in ten years" line and sits down on the floor. I stop searching for the cap and sit down next to her. Rolling the needle between my fingers, I apologize again.

I try to be more careful now, replacing the orange cap and throwing the syringe into the trash can across the room. The needles are as aerodynamic as a spear, and I can hit almost any target with them. They're like an extension of my finger. I close one eye, position my fingers around the needle, take aim, and release it forward. I rarely miss the plastic trash can between the desks in our room.

I don't tell my mom about Angie sitting on the needle when she calls, because I know she'll mail me another Planters Peanut jar. She sent three with me when I moved up here, telling me I had to be considerate of others. No one wants to look at needles lying around a room. It's not like our house, my mom said. She packed insulin to keep in our dorm refrigerator and enough needles to last me for months. No one here knows I'm diabetic, and I don't tell them. My mom insisted on notifying my floor monitor and wrote a letter to the girl. I told my mom I'd give it to her, but I threw it away. The professors don't even know my name, let alone anything about my illness. I'm thankful that I'm not like the girl in the wheelchair in my English class. Visible disability. It's easy to hide my illness up here.

I CHOOSE English as my major the second semester. My sister gave me Kahlil Gibran's *The Prophet* when I graduated from high school, and I want to express myself on paper like he does. I repeat the poem "On Children" over and over under my breath as I walk to class. I want to read books, talk about literature, do something I enjoy. I started as a computer science major, and Angie told me to stop being so practical. "Don't worry about the future," she says. "Do what you want."

I call Denise to tell her my decision. When she says poetry will make me happy, I hear the distance in her voice. I wrap my fingers around the telephone receiver and envision her curled up on the couch in her house. I can hear the television playing in the background. She says she's fine, busy at work. I want to tell her that I miss home, miss her. Instead I tell her the story about Angie sitting on my needle. I want to hear her laugh, but she doesn't. She tells me it was pretty stupid to leave a needle sticking in the couch. She's lost her sense of humor. She sounds preoccupied, nervous.

I call her more often. Sometimes she doesn't answer, but I know she's there. When I hear the beep of the answering machine, I tell her to pick up. Then I wait. I envision her staring at the telephone, hand paused in midair above the receiver. I want to talk to her. Summer is almost here, and I'm thinking about moving back to Des Moines to live next year. Angie and I aren't getting along anymore, and the girls on my floor are all busy with boyfriends now. I decide leaving campus is the best idea. I want to be closer to my parents and Denise. I can commute the forty miles to class next year.

The red numbers of the digital alarm clock glare against the blackness of my bedroom. 1:51 A.M. Fighting to keep my eyes open for a moment longer, I listen for the sound that startled me from sleep. Silence. I tell myself it's just the sound of a house I'm not familiar with. I know my sister was asleep when I went to bed. Just as my eyelids start to close again, I hear the sound of glass crunching against the linoleum floor in the kitchen. My body freezes for several seconds before I scramble out of bed. I turn the corner to the hallway and see her on the floor in the kitchen. She's flat on her back and her head is tilted toward me. The refrigerator door is open, and the dim light from inside casts shadows onto my sister's pale skin. A glass pitcher has shattered around her motionless body, and orange juice stains the front of her nightgown. Wiping the sleep from my eyes, I jump up the three steps to the kitchen and kneel beside her.

"Are you awake?" I ask, shaking her shoulder. "Denise, wake up."

A soft groan escapes her lips.

I know what to do. I yank open the cabinet door and grab candy from the shelf. I place a peppermint pinwheel under her tongue and speak firmly to her.

"Wake up, Denise. Suck on the candy."

I push her bent leg flat to the ground and close the refrigerator door. Carefully moving the shattered glass away from her dark hair, I set my hand against the side of her face. Her cheek is sweaty and cold. As I get up to flip on the kitchen light, a jagged piece of glass cuts into my knee. I reach down and pull the glass from my skin. Blood runs down the front of my leg. My sister's eyelashes flutter. She opens her eyes wide and stares at the ceiling.

"What an ordeal, huh?" she mumbles.

Several minutes pass before I inch closer to her.

She pushes her body into a sitting position and looks down at the glass surrounding her. I let all the air out of my lungs, and watch her eyes move around the room as she tries to piece together what has happened. With her back against the refrigerator, she wipes drops of orange juice from her face and neck with the back of her hand. I pull a granola bar from the cabinet and place it in her hand. Her thin fingers grasp the plastic wrapper.

I don't have to ask what happened, but she starts to explain anyway. She talks slowly.

"I crawled to the kitchen and thought I could pour the orange juice from the top shelf into my mouth. It just fell." She looks down at the mess again. "It was like a waterfall and then the pitcher came crashing down."

"Why don't you put some candy by your bed, Denise?"

She gives me a blank stare.

"One of these times I'm not going to hear you out here, and I'm going to wake up and you're going to be in a coma."

I'm annoyed. This is the third time I've found her like this in the last two months. Her blood sugar plummets while she's sleeping, and I wonder what she did before I moved in. She reminds me that she was just fine living on her own.

"Whatever, Denise," I reply, dismissing her irritated tone as the low blood sugar speaking. "We'll talk about it tomorrow."

She closes her eyes and leans her head against the refrigerator door.

I know the feeling of waking up at three A.M. and barely being able to move. My blood sugar sometimes gets too low when I'm sleeping, and I try to convince myself I can sleep through it until morning. The heaviness of sleep combined with the lack of energy from low blood sugar is hard to overcome. I know how she feels. I've had to force myself out of bed some nights too. But the difference is that I get up and go to the kitchen and she waits until it's too late.

"I wish you would make yourself get out of bed instead of closing your eyes again," I tell her.

The innocent, empty expression on her face makes me shudder.

"I'm just afraid sometime you might not wake up," I tell her. My voice is apologetic now.

"I always wake up, Andie," she replies, wrapping her fingers around the refrigerator door handle. The sleeves on her night-gown are short and the fibers of her muscles seem to push through her flesh. Her arm is too thin. She pulls herself up and looks down at the stained nightgown and shakes her head. "I always wake up," she repeats.

"I'm not trying to be your mother," I tell her. "It just seems like you're not taking care of yourself."

"I'm fine," she replies, still annoyed.

I follow Denise down the long hallway to her bedroom. She turns on the television before crawling under the covers. I sit down on the bed next to her. Sometimes I sleep in here. We watch movies late into the night and fall asleep with the television on. She loves comedies, and her copies of *Coming to America* and *A Fish Called Wanda* sit on top of the dresser. She watches them over and over, laughing just as hard each time. She can stay in bed and watch comedies for hours on the weekend. With a burning cigarette dangling from her fingers, she recites the lines along with the television.

The voice of a late-night talk-show host fills the room as Denise flips over on her stomach and cradles the pillow under her chin. I pick up the remote control from the nightstand and turn the volume down. The lips of the comedian being interviewed on television open and close enthusiastically, but no sound escapes the screen. Denise mumbles something in her sleep and repositions her body under the covers. Turning her back to me, she curls into a ball and her breathing evens out. I know she won't remember any of this in the morning.

She always forgets what has happened when she gets like this. Insulin is looking for sugar in her body, depriving the nervous system and cerebral cortex of energy. The result is disorientation and memory loss. She won't remember the insulin reaction or talking to me. Going to bed will be the last thing she remembers when she wakes up in the morning. I won't remind her of what happened tonight.

She's always been a heavy sleeper. When I was a kid, my brother and I made a game out of trying to wake her up. We tickled her toes and slowly inched the covers off her half-clothed body. One morning my brother and I sneaked in and set an ice cube on her chest. We fell to the floor, holding our stomachs and trying to contain our laughter. We expected her to wake up but finally grew bored waiting for the ice cube to melt. The pool of water ran down onto her nightgown and she never stirred. When we finally resorted to pouring a glass of cold water on her forehead, she installed a lock on her bedroom door.

I was only six then, but I remember her arguing with my mother over the dead bolt. My mom still checked on Denise in the middle of the night, sat next to her bed and listened to her breathing. She'd been doing that Denise's whole life. My mother tried to convince Denise that it wasn't safe to have a door that locked with little kids in the house. But the lock stayed, and some nights I would hear my mother in the hallway outside Denise's bedroom. Her slippers shuffled back and forth on the hardwood floor.

My mother worried because one morning a year earlier, Denise didn't wake up. It was a Saturday in early May and my family was getting ready to go to a wedding when the phone rang. It was my sister's friend Robin. I told her Denise was still asleep, but Robin said it was important, so I knocked on Denise's door. No response. I started to pound, annoyed that she was ignoring me. My brother rushed by, speaking into a walkie-talkie to the boy who lived next door. My mom was packing her suitcase in the bedroom downstairs, and my dad was out in the garage. I knocked a few more times and finally opened the door. My sister was on her stomach with the sheet pulled halfway up her back. I yelled at her from the doorway, but she didn't respond.

At this point my mother's story differs from mine. My mom says that she came into the room, turned Denise over, and found that the bed was wet. Denise had peed in her sleep. My mother says she started screaming for me to call the ambulance, but I didn't move. I remember turning Denise over myself. The smell of urine was strong, and her body was heavy beneath my small hands. I remember being frozen, unable to move from beside the bed to call for help. My mother just appeared in the doorway and approached the bed to see what had happened. I remember it so well because I thought my sister was dead. My mom was crying and my sister wouldn't wake up and my brother lingered in the doorway, looking like he was going to cry too. My dad was outside in the garage, and time stopped next to Denise's bed.

The ambulance wailed down the street, and the men in white picked my sister up and put her on a gurney. Her leg fell limp over the side, and one of the men pushed it back onto the thin mattress and secured the straps across her legs and chest. My parents wouldn't let me go to the hospital with them. I had to stay with my neighbor, an old, nosy woman who kept asking me questions about my sister's diabetes. I waited all day at her house for the phone to ring. When my parents finally returned, they said Denise had amnesia. Hopefully, it would be temporary. My sister couldn't remember her own name, said she didn't know my mom and dad. The doctors told my parents she would come around. Diabetic comas sometimes cause memory loss.

Denise came home the next day, but her memory hadn't completely returned. When she walked in the front door with my father, she looked around the living room like it wasn't familiar. She stared at me for several seconds before smiling at me like I was just a cute little girl, not anyone she knew. Not her sister. In the days that followed, she would forget to give her shots, or else she would give one and then give another one five minutes later. My dad hid her insulin and only gave it to her when he knew she was going to eat. She kept asking my mother what had happened, why she wasn't going to school.

My parents told her the story over and over. She looked at them like she didn't believe their words. I remember sitting in a restaurant with my family about a week after the incident. I was eating a grilled cheese but staring at my mother's pork tenderloin. Denise started with the questions again, asking why she had gone to the hospital. My dad laughed and told her to look in her pocket. He had typed up a sheet of the events and given it to her earlier that day. He was tired of answering her questions. My sister looked down at the pocket on her T-shirt and reached inside. She looked surprised at the existence of the white piece of paper and unfolded it slowly. She read it, nodded her head, and folded it back up before returning it to her pocket.

My dad laughs when he tells this story now. He says the amnesia that followed was funny only because he knew Denise was going to be okay. My mom's voice still cracks when she talks about that day. She says we could have easily left for the wedding and never checked on my sister. Denise would have been dead by the time we returned the next day. My mom has spent her life worrying about whether or not my sister is going to wake up in the morning.

Now I worry about Denise. Sometimes I find myself checking on her in the middle of the night. I think my parents are relieved we're living together. My mother doesn't worry so much. Her daughters take care of each other now. I look down at my sister. She's snoring.

I remember the broken glass in the kitchen, and I slide my bare feet into my sister's slippers on the floor. We wear the same size shoes. After moving into her house, I was excited to find that I could wear her black leather boots in the winter. I have been waiting for years to grow into her shoes.

I walk slowly down the dark hall, brushing my fingers lightly along the wall as I go. My heart is still beating hard as I step into the empty kitchen. Pulling a dishrag from the sink, I bend down and push the shattered glass into a pile on the linoleum. Tiny, sharp spears poke through the thin material into my fingers, and the orange juice soaks the white rag. The hem of my long white T-shirt is stained with the juice. I open the refrigerator door and wipe orange drops from the plastic shelves.

It's a new refrigerator. My sister ordered it two weeks ago. The old one made popping sounds and didn't keep the ice frozen. Denise stood smiling in the middle of the kitchen when the delivery men wheeled it through the door. I thought she was going to kiss the young boy in the baseball cap when he pushed it into the corner. It's shiny and clean and looks out of place in the old kitchen. The other appliances are gold, reminiscent of the seventies. Denise wants to tear up the floor and rip out the cupboards in here. She desires a new kitchen with bright white countertops. The refrigerator is the first piece of her dream room.

Orange juice has spilled down into the fruit drawers, and I pull them out and turn them upside down in the dishwasher. Pushing the rag into the back corners of the refrigerator, I wipe away the evidence of tonight. I wipe signs of the struggle from the plastic shelves. Then I pull a can of frozen orange juice from the freezer and place it on the top shelf of the refrigerator to thaw.

After running cold water over my hands, I rinse and fold the dishrag and walk back to Denise's bedroom. Her brown hair wraps around her face, and her lips form words in her sleep. I look around the bedroom. Clothes are strewn around the floor, and glasses half full of water are sweating on the furniture. Her college diplomas are framed and hanging on the wall. Pictures of friends are glued to the mirror on her dresser. Most of her girlfriends have gotten married and have children. Scenes from my sister's life flash in front of me as I slide the slippers off my feet and crawl under the covers next to her.

I close my eyes and try to relax, but my adrenaline is still flowing. My heart pounds from the fear I felt almost an hour ago. A fear that was born that morning in her bedroom when I was five years old. The fear that my sister is going to die. I try to make my body relax. Listening to Denise breathe, I make my own breath match the inhales and exhales. In and out. Slow and measured.

Three Days

Denise's car is parked in the driveway and the house is dark. The sun has fallen too far below the trees to cast shadows on single objects, but the whole house seems to be shrouded in a dark shadow of its own. The sky is a fading violet. I look through the windshield of my car at our empty garbage can next to the street. A stiff wind rocks it back and forth.

My eyes are glued to the dark living room window as I get out of my car and walk slowly toward the porch. I've been out of town for three days, and there is an eerie silence about the house that makes my heart pound. The streetlights illuminate the unmowed grass in front of the house, and though I suddenly feel almost paralyzed with fear, something pushes me forward to the front door. I test the doorknob. Locked. I don't insert my key. Instead I step away from the door like a worried neighbor who knows something isn't right but doesn't feel she has the authority to enter the house uninvited. I'm going to look in the windows.

I'm overreacting. I should just go in. My sister is probably out with a friend. Someone must have picked her up for a movie and she forgot to turn the porch light on. Maybe she fell asleep on the couch in the living room. I look like a prowler, sneaking around out here. Denise and I will really get a laugh if the old woman next door calls the police on me. But I can't talk my heart into slowing its beat. I raise myself up on my tiptoes and press my face against the glass. The living room is dark except for shadows of familiar furniture and red dots on the stereo. Straining to make out a shape curled up on the couch or floor, I squint my eyes. Nothing. I walk around the outside of the house, looking in each window for some sign of my sister. As I approach one of the windows to her room, I take a deep breath, thinking of something my mother once told me. If there was a heated argument between the next-door neighbors or an ambulance pulled up across the street, my mother would turn out the lights inside the house before going to the window. *They can't see you looking out if the lights are off,* she told me. She was right. I can barely make out the shapes of Denise's bed and dresser. Warm summer wind blows against the hairs on the back of my neck.

Relief spreads over me as I push my key into the lock on the front door. I'm being ridiculous. I would have noticed if something was really wrong inside the house, but turning the doorknob, I think of the bathroom. It was the only room I couldn't see into from where I stood outside. I reach my hand inside the front door and flip a switch. The light is bright in the living room now, shining through the windows onto the grass outside. Everything is in place. A mechanical clack makes me jump. The CD player is changing a disc, but the volume has been turned all the way down. The red Repeat light is flashing. The six discs inside will play over and over until someone turns the stereo off. I turn the volume up. The voice of Billy Joel in his younger days fills the room. "Travelin' Prayer." A blanket is folded neatly on the couch, and the answering machine light is blinking. A novel my sister has been reading rests facedown and open on the arm of our favorite overstuffed chair.

The air in here is still and stale. I don't yell for my sister. Dropping my suitcase and keys to the floor, I walk down the hall. My bedroom and the den are undisturbed. As I make my way down the hallway toward the bathroom, goose bumps form on my arms. My shoulders tighten as I reach for the light switch. Empty. The white tile on the floor sparkles and a towel has been thrown onto the rug. I exhale loudly and pick up the terry-cloth towel. Denise never remembers to hang it up. I check the toilet because it smells in here. Bright white and sparkling. The faucet is dripping and toothpaste is stuck to the drain in the sink. I catch a glimpse of myself in the mirror. I study my reflection and try to blink the fear out of my eyes.

I curl my hand around the doorknob on the other end of the bathroom. I entered through the hallway door, but the second door leads to my sister's bedroom. The light from the bathroom casts a peach-gray glow across her dark carpet. My sister is on the bed. She is flat on her stomach and her head is tilted toward me. Her eyes are open and her face is bloated. She looks plastic and inhuman. One swollen arm is sprawled across the mattress, fingers outstretched. She has tucked the other arm under her chest. A bare foot dangles toward the floor and her legs look as though they have been pumped full of fluid. She is limp like a neglected doll. A fan in the window blows hot, humid air against her dark hair, producing the only movement in the room.

My knees shake uncontrollably, and my gaze shifts to the window I looked through only moments before. I brace my arms on either side of the doorway to support the sudden heaviness of my back. I need to get to my sister. As I inch my way onto the carpet in her bedroom, death envelops me. My body is moving on its own. I bend down and touch her cheek, expecting to feel icy, cold death, but the room is too hot. She is cool and damp. The lyrics to "Piano Man" drift down the hallway. Cars pass on the street outside and a telephone rings across the darkness of the neighborhood. The air feels thick as I sit down on the bed next to her and lock my eyes with hers.

I don't know how much time passes before I pick up the telephone and call the police. But once I hang up the receiver, it seems like only seconds before I hear the sirens. Then the pounding on the door. I had only reported to the 911 operator that there was a dead body in the house. Then I hung up. Men in suits arrive. The detectives hover around the room, glancing occasionally at each other with somber eyes before trying to politely snap pictures of the corpse. They scribble on notepads and talk into tape recorders. The unexplainable, sudden death of a thirty-three-year-old woman makes them curious. They walk through every room of the house, looking for signs of forced entry or foul play. They find nothing, and no one touches her until the coroner arrives. He towers over her bed and pronounces her dead. Makes it official.

Then they start asking me questions. Was she on drugs? Did she have health problems? Had she been alone in the house? How long had I been on vacation? Who was the last person to see her alive? When had I talked to her last? I look up from my spot at the kitchen table and silently stare at them, as if they are speaking a foreign language. I study the faces of each of the men, but I can't speak. I want them to leave. There are too many people in our kitchen. I want to be alone with my sister again.

I'm not answering their questions, but they aren't angry with me. One of the men tells me I'm in shock and says he understands. Finally, a female officer in uniform picks up Denise's purse off the kitchen counter. My sister always sets her bag in the same spot, next to the canisters marked "Sugar" and "Flour." The officer rummages through it while the others watch. Her eyes narrow and she looks up at me before pulling a vial of white powder from the side pocket of the bag. Cocaine. Her search also uncovers prescription sedatives, needles, and insulin. The detectives seem satisfied.

My parents appear in the doorway. Tears have stained my mother's cheeks. She has been crying in the car. My father's eyes drift slowly across the room, finally falling on me at the kitchen table surrounded by officers. He puts his hand on my mother's shoulder. She's hysterical now and insists on seeing her daughter. Her other daughter. A detective tells her maybe she should just sit in the living room, but my mom pushes past him and runs down the hall. Her high-pitched moan breaks the silence in the house. My father disappears down the hallway after her.

The detectives have temporarily stopped questioning me, and I stand up. I should be with my parents, I tell myself. The family should all be in the bedroom together. I make my way down the hall and find my mother on the floor next to the bathroom door. My father is slumped on the rocking chair watching as the investigators take pictures of the scene. They have pulled her swelled head away from her pillow, exposing a brown stain beneath. Her skin is purplish and looks as though it has melted from her bones. My father's voice cracks when he asks one of the paramedics how long she's been dead. Three days, at least, the man in blue replies. Rigor mortis has set in and settled out. He goes on to explain that when the heart stops beating, blood settles outward to the skin, particularly in the area bearing the weight of the body. Because my sister had been lying on her stomach, the blood was pushed forward into her face. The man in blue waves his arm around my sister's body like a college professor as he explains the process of death to my father. I stare at my family. My mother on the floor with her head buried in her arms. My father staring intently at the man in blue explaining why my sister no longer looks human. My sister, eyes still open, watching us all.

MY MIND is free from the image of my sister's body when I wake up the morning of her funeral. I hit the button on my alarm clock and feel a brief moment of relief. Somewhere between deep sleep and the last nap before waking, my mind is clear. I have been dreaming about an African vacation where I was riding on a bus with my friends and the colors of the animals leaped out at me. The dream was peaceful, and as I reach for the alarm clock, I cling to the image of open fields and clear skies. Then I blink my eyes several times and the weight on my chest returns. The image of her face burns in my head.

The responsibility of burying my sister belongs to me. I picked out the plot and casket yesterday. Pulling clothes from her closet and delivering them to the mortician was my duty. I spoke to the coroner about his failure to rule on the cause of death. He insisted on an autopsy and I nodded in agreement. The decision to have a closed-casket funeral was mine. The man at the funeral home told me he could put some color back into her face, but I shook my head as I stared across the counter at him. I knew I couldn't look at her again.

I ride to the funeral with my family. A long black limousine pulls up to my parents' house, and the neighbors stare as we file into the car. The solemn-faced driver maneuvers through the streets slowly and carefully, as if the speed of the car should match our mood. Finally, he pulls up to the white stone building. The sun burns through my black hat as I walk from the limousine to the front door. I step into the lobby and am overwhelmed by the smell of flowers. It makes me sick.

A black and white board to my left lists the surnames of the people who have died and the rooms their bodies are in. Ahead of me there is a steep staircase. There are more rooms upstairs, and I'm thankful they've placed Denise on the ground level. I don't think I could make it up to the top right now. I look at the board. My sister is listed simply "Dominick—3." When I chose her spot at the cemetery, my parents bought their own as well. Actually, my dad ended up paying for four plots in a row on the top of the little grassy hill. I might not get married either.

I step into the rented room. A wreath of orchids rests on top of the silver casket. Two banners hang from the center. The words "Sister" and "Daughter" are printed in pink, and the oblong box is skirted with a crisp white cloth. The casket looks like it belongs here in this room. Frozen in time. A collage of photographs of my sister and our family rests on a stand in the corner. My brother dug through picture albums and boxes yesterday to put it together. I sit down on a padded chair in the corner of the pale pink room and force my eyes away from the casket. It's too finely polished, too expensive. This place looks like someone's living room. The ceiling is spackled. A small, cheap stereo hides behind a lamp on a table. Yesterday the man here told me I could make my own tapes for the visitation. He thought I might like to play my sister's favorite songs. The idea of George Thorogood wailing in my grandmother's ears almost made me laugh. I wanted to ask him if people danced at these events, but I just shook my head. Play whatever you usually play, I told the man.

My brother leans against the wall next to the door. He's gained at least twenty pounds since I saw him last, and his suit jacket rests on either side of his stomach. He's been gone so long. I don't know him anymore. He is married now, and he and his wife are trying to have kids. I want to put my hand on his shoulder and remind him that now we're a family with only two siblings. The desire to touch my brother is overwhelming. He is the only family I have left—the only family with a chance of living as long as I do. My parents are in their sixties. They will die before their children. Or so I had thought. I have always accepted that as the natural progression of life. My mother and father will leave, and I will be left with my siblings. I thought my sister would at least outlive my father. I press my back against the chair and study my brother carefully.

My mother hovers near the casket the entire morning. She has aged ten years in two days. Her hair contains more strands of gray, and wrinkles have formed beneath her swollen eyes. She is constantly surrounded by people, feeling the obligation to play the part of the hostess at a gathering. She occasionally glances at my father who sits alone on a pastel floral couch against the wall. He talks to no one and stares out the window.

The four of us stay separated in this room. I am grateful for the presence of the visitors. They give my family safety from the fear each of us has that we will break down if we have to speak to each other. I am fine as long as I avoid looking at my father. Most of the morning I stare at my new shoes. They have a two-inch heel and cause the ball of my foot to ache. I have never worn heels for more than a few minutes at a time before today. Whenever I tried them on in a store, I always found them uncomfortable, unnecessary. Ann convinced me to buy these painful black shoes yesterday. She said they were appropriate for the occasion.

Now I want to take the shoes off. I want to take them off and stretch out on the couch next to my father and put my head in his lap. I would let him stroke my brown hair the way he did when I was a little girl. And we could go back in time to the days when we were a family with three kids. But I don't move. I just stare at my shoes and twist my feet around on the mauve carpet.

My sister always wore high heels. I picked out her favorite gray four-inchers to bury her in. When I handed them to the mortician, I wondered if he would stuff her swollen feet into the narrow shoes or simply rest them against her ankles in the bottom of the casket. Denise always loved the shoes that made her five-foot-four-inch frame seem taller. She had a pair to match every outfit and always claimed her feet were comfortable. I tried several times over the years to fit my feet into my sister's heels and walk normally. She would sit on the edge of her bed and laugh, telling me she had seen drag queens that looked more graceful than I did.

I FINALLY take my shoes off at the cemetery. I slipped my feet halfway out of them as the minister spoke during the service, but I never completely removed them. In the back of the limousine on the way here, I rubbed my ankles and the tops of my feet but forced myself to suffer. Now, as the casket hovers above the grave, I finally reach down and pull the shoes off by the heels. I stand next to Ann, feeling the cool grass between my toes. I am lost in the comfort of physical relief, and I close my eyes as the minister's monotone voice drones in the background.

Several minutes pass before I open my eyes to the polite stirring of people. The service has ended and they are heading for their cars. They step carefully as they make their way down the hill. No one wants to walk on the grass above the spot where a casket might be buried. I stand alone, face-to-face with the minister. Not wanting to meet his eyes, I scan the green cemetery. A man is leaning against a pickup truck on the other side of the hill. He's waiting for us to leave. A strange urge comes over me. I leave my shoes nestled in the grass and run for him. I know I am a strange sight to people who turn to watch. The dead woman's sister has finally lost it, they think. I stop when I reach the man leaning against the truck.

"Will you please lower the casket?" I ask, catching my breath.

He gives me a perplexed look.

"Please," I plead.

"Well, uh, I usually wait until everyone is gone, miss."

I look down at my bare feet and twirl my toes around in a circle in the grass, like if I stand there long enough he will feel sorry for me and change his mind. Finally, he turns and walks toward the grave. I follow him, trailing several feet behind. He looks at me and then down to the road at the retreating guests. He stares at the casket for a moment before resting his hand on the crank that will lower the oblong box. It disappears beneath the ground and he steps back, hoping this is satisfactory. I look down at my feet again to let him know I need to see more. He throws a shovelful of dirt down into the hole. I hear the earth hit metal, and I turn and walk toward the limousine.

The limousine driver steps out and opens the door for me. I look at the man shoveling dirt. I want to run back and pull the casket up with my own hands. Grab my sister from it and wake her up. I need my sister, but the driver is staring at me. His black hat casts a shadow over his face. He's probably late for his next appointment, so I lower my body into the black car and rest my head on my father's shoulder. My dad's hand shakes as he reaches over to pat my thigh. The driver shuts the door.

Numb

I SHUT DOWN completely after the funeral. I won't leave my house. The sun beats down on the pavement outside and the humidity in the air settles on my skin, but I remain on the floor with my legs stretched out beneath the coffee table. I rest my back against the front of the couch and stare at the television. It's been tuned to the same channel all week. Sometimes I watch the dust on the furniture, the way the sun glares through the windows and bounces off it. Week-old glasses of lemonade leave rings on the hardwood floor around me, and the ashtray is overflowing. I smoke the Marlboro Reds Denise left behind. I ignore the irritation in my throat caused by the hot smoke. The burning cigarette smells like my sister. The smoke circles around my face and stings my eyes. But I don't blink.

The day before the funeral, I pulled all my sister's belongings from her bedroom into the living room. Now boxes are piled on the floor between the television set and where I sit. I emptied her dresser drawers into piles against the walls, and I stare at the television over crates marked "Texts," "Thesis," and "Old T-shirts." The clothes from her closet are on hangers over the backs of chairs, and her bedroom furniture fills the once-empty space in the living room. Her possessions surround me, but I barely notice them.

Outside my windows, the neighborhood is alive with children on summer vacation. Bikes skid to a stop on the sidewalk in front of my house, and the familiar cries of scraped knees and elbows ring through the air. Softballs bounce in my driveway. The roar of my neighbor's lawn mower drifts through my windows, and the smell of cut grass follows. Mothers call their children in for dinner. The days are long and sticky and distantly familiar. Lives move forward on the streets outside my house.

I'm never fully aware of my isolation until the afternoons when I hear my father's car pull into my driveway. It's the same scene every day. I push myself up onto the couch and run my fingers through my unwashed hair. I grab the remote control from between the cushions of the couch and turn up the volume on the television. I place a magazine in my lap and take a deep breath as my father turns the doorknob on the front door.

"Hi there," he says, his voice shaking.

I raise my hand in return. I have stopped speaking. My dad doesn't take it personally. He walks into the room that resembles a forgotten attic, and looks around at the clutter.

"Do you want to get some lunch?" he asks.

I shake my head.

"A bike ride?" he says, trying to elicit some response from me.

A bike ride? I wonder.

But I don't respond. After the funeral, I planned on going back to work at my part-time summer job right away, told myself I had to keep moving to get on with my life, but I had a breakdown. I started to cry and couldn't stop. That lasted for two days, and now I've been sitting on my living room floor for five more. I can't find the energy to move.

My dad puts his hand on my shoulder and reminds me that I could use a shower.

Anger stirs in my chest, but I say nothing. I know he's right. My body is sticky from dried sweat, and I haven't washed my hair since the morning of the funeral. I've been wearing my sister's *Far Side* T-shirt. The cartoon on the front is of a boy pushing on a door that says PULL. The sign above him reads,

MIDVILLE SCHOOL FOR THE GIFTED. Denise loved *The Far Side*. When I touch my face, my fingers are met with dried tears and oily grime.

"Holly and Ann say you're not answering the phone," he tells me on this, the fifth day. "They've been calling our house wondering if you're all right."

I look over at the phone. It's been ringing, and I've been ignoring it. I think about my friends. Holly drove me everywhere the day before the funeral. She took me to the mall to find a black dress and to the cemetery to pick out a plot. I avoided my family. I spent time with Ann and Holly because they didn't remind me of Denise. They weren't grieving. I didn't have to comfort them like I thought I did my parents. I welcomed their presence until the afternoon Denise's body was lowered into the ground. Now I don't want to see anyone. But being around my friends would be easier than facing my dad every day. I don't know what to say to him.

Neither of us is ready to talk about Denise, and I think somehow he's relieved that I'm so silent day after day. If we don't talk, we won't cry. I've never really seen my dad cry, and I don't know how I'd handle it if he did. But I feel guilty for not acknowledging him. I know he's lonely. My mother probably doesn't talk to him either. I imagine her rushing around the kitchen every night preparing dinner. Then placing a plate for my dad on the table and retreating to her bedroom. We all wait for the shock to wear off.

Each day when he arrives at my house, he looks around the living room to see if anything has changed, searches for a sign that I'm going to snap out of my isolation. He tries to get me to talk by asking simple questions, but I won't respond. He brings pots of spaghetti or potato salad that my mother has prepared and places them in the refrigerator, surely noticing that I haven't touched what he left the day before. Then he wanders around my kitchen for a few minutes, rinsing out a glass or wiping down the already-clean counter. Finally he sits down next to me on the couch and pretends to watch whatever is on the television.

I don't look over at him as he leans against the armrest on the opposite end of the couch. Focusing on the television, we sit still, pretend the tension surrounding us doesn't exist. After about thirty minutes, he stands up to leave. As he walks toward the door, he reaches down and squeezes my shoulder again and tells me to call if I need anything. I want to place my hand on his, but I can't move. When he opens the door to leave, fresh summer air rushes in. Then he hesitates before closing the door behind him. Tears run down my cheeks as he starts up his car and backs down the driveway. And just when I hear him accelerate down the street and away from my house, I want him back. I cry more because I have said nothing to him. I am alone and I am pushing him away.

My behavior scares me. I'm aware of my distance, and my biggest fear is that I'll never return to normal. I'll never stop feeling this way. I won't know how to be the person I used to be. I lie in bed at night and stare at the ceiling, pretending it's a month earlier. Trying to remember what I felt like before she died. I can't. I have no sense of what my life was like before last week. I think maybe I never possessed an identity of my own, and I won't be able to find myself again without my sister.

I lose my awareness of time. Sometimes I pace the house at two in the morning and sleep six or seven hours during the day. The only thing I know is that it's three o'clock in the afternoon when my father arrives each day. His presence reminds me that the rest of the world is moving on as I sit on my living room floor. But then the sun drops and the crickets chirp and I am alone in the dark again.

I hate the dark now. Nightmares plague me after the sun sets. I have dreams that my sister is standing above me while I sleep. Her skin looks like it's rotting, and her eyes are hollow. She tells me over and over that she just wants to talk. I tell her to go away, but she won't leave. I force myself to wake up, but then I'm afraid to open my eyes. I think she's going to be right there, pissed that I've pulled all her possessions into the living room. I can't breathe and sharp pain shoots through my chest. Fear paralyzes me. Sometimes it's so bad I close my eyes tight, curl up against the couch, and wait until three o'clock when my father arrives. Unable to move, I wait hours until I hear his car door slam. Then I force myself to sit up.

Images of my sister snorting cocaine plague me. I was in junior high the first time I saw her use the drug. I walked into the bedroom of her house and saw her inhaling the white powder. Her back was to me, but I watched her reflection in the mirror. She tapped a razor blade against the oak dresser and formed lines with the white dust. Then she picked up a rolled dollar bill and leaned down. She inhaled. Once. Twice. Smoke from the cigarette burning in the ashtray surrounded her head, danced in her hair. I backed slowly out of the room. She didn't know I'd seen her, and I buried the memory, convinced myself it had been a dream.

When I moved into this house, I spotted the vials and razor blades on her dresser right away. Small envelopes made from magazine paper lined the oak top. Some were still folded. Others had been opened up and licked clean. I was older, and Denise didn't try to hide her habit. She talked about cocaine like it was television. Something to do. I wasn't surprised that she knew everything about the drug. She had kits to test for quality, screens to sift the white powder, vials, tooters, mirrors, and razor blades. Lots of razor blades. She explained to me that magazine paper was the best choice for packaging cocaine. It doesn't absorb moisture, the ink doesn't run, and she could lick every last granule off it. It is easy, cheap, and disposable.

My curiosity got the best of me, and on my twentieth birthday I tried the drug. My sister watched me closely as I pulled a rock from the envelope and placed it on the top of a small screen. I rubbed it through onto the mirror on the dresser. My hands shook and I inhaled. I threw my head back and sniffed hard. It burned my nose, but I did the second line immediately. Anyone watching me would have thought I'd done it a hundred times. Warmth rushed over me and my eyes opened wide. I ran my finger across the mirror and picked up the remaining granules. I did everything the way I'd seen Denise do it. It seemed instinctual. I smoothed white powder over my teeth and gums. They went numb. I immediately understood her addiction. I understood the lab monkeys I'd read about in psychology class who refused food for another fix. I sat down on my sister's bed and watched her snort lines. We talked and smoked all night, and when I wasn't smoking, I played with Denise's Zippo lighter. Taking it apart and putting it back together. Checking the flint again and again.

I did cocaine because of Denise. That's what I told myself anyway. It was something we shared, something we did together, something we didn't tell our parents about. I was excited. Then excitement turned to nervousness after a few weeks. I started losing too much weight. My nose burned and my back hurt and I knew I had too much to lose. It was the first time my nature dominated my desire to be like my sister. I never did the drug again. I couldn't live my sister's life, but I rationalized that she was different. I accepted her. Cocaine forced me to understand unconditional love.

She wasn't the stereotypical addict. She was just Denise. She got up for work every day and relaxed with novels at night. I told myself she had her life under control. Now I know she was self-destructive. She had a subconscious desire to take her own life before diabetes did. Smoking and drinking in excess throughout her twenties and rarely visiting the doctor, she frequently ran out of insulin and needles and never tested her blood sugars. Her only motivation to exercise was to stay thin, and she sometimes wouldn't eat for days. Even though she never weighed more than 115 pounds, she thought she was fat and smoked cigarettes to calm the rumbling in her stomach. It's clear to me now as I sit surrounded by her things. She always thought the disease would kill her eventually anyway. She grew up knowing what would take her life. Denise laughed and said she wished she would live long enough to die from lung cancer. She didn't.

I close my eyes and force myself to search for happy memories. I remember the way she protected me when I was growing up and insisted I start thinking about college before I even got to high school. I remember the way her arms reached confidently in front of her when she received her M.A. in psychology from Drake University. I recall the way she ran her finger across the base of her nose and sniffed. Her hair in curlers and a cigarette dangling from her lips as she prepared herself for an evening out. How her body had been stretched across her bed the night I found her. She becomes too real to me now.

NINE DAYS after I bury my sister, I slide myself from my spot on the couch onto the floor and open a cardboard box labeled "Pictures." I pull a worn photo album from the box onto my lap. As I open the first page, my sister smiles at me. She is standing in a swimsuit with her friend Gail in front of a boat. The sun is beating down on her shoulders and she's holding a can of beer. I remember her stories about this trip. Denise fell asleep in the Florida sun on the first day of her vacation and got a bad sunburn. Her body looks stiff in the picture, like she's afraid if she moves, the pain of the sunburn will sting her. But her eyes are laughing.

I turn the pages, amazed at how happy she looks in all the snapshots. Photographs from parties and vacations and days at the beach. I stop when I come to a picture of me standing next to her. The two of us are leaning against a tree, tilting our heads together. I was about fifteen and I remember the trip well. She took me camping in Arkansas for the weekend with several of her friends. She let me try a beer and I spit it into the campfire. Instead of laughing at me, she reached into the cooler and pulled out a can of pop. This picture was taken the next morn ing after we crawled out of the tent. Our clothes were wrinkled and my hair was sticking up all around my head. Her friend Kent told us to stand in front of the tree and make funny faces. Neither of us did. We are facing the camera and smiling, but her eyes are gazing at me.

I stare at the picture for the longest time, lost in the feeling that she is alive. Studying the details of our faces, I see the strong resemblance that so many people have commented on. I was taller than her, a fact Denise attributed to her getting diabetes earlier in life than I did, but we looked alike. I peel the picture from the sticky page of the album and stand up. Holding it carefully between my thumb and forefinger, I extend my arm and hold it up level with my eyes. Looking down at my own legs and then back to the picture, I think about how much older I am getting.

A bead of sweat runs down my cheek and dangles at the bottom of my jaw. The heat that has been weighing on me for days suddenly makes me restless. My heart throbs against my chest. I look around the messy living room with wonder. It's like I'm noticing it for the first time. My sister's life stares back at me.

I turn away from the boxes and walk down the hall toward the bathroom, pausing only briefly in the doorway of my sister's empty bedroom. Standing in front of the full-length mirror behind the bathroom door, I hold the photograph next to my face and look from the picture to myself over and over. I am close to the same age now that she was in the picture. My face is the same rounded shape, and my thin, brown hair falls over my shoulders like hers did. I stare at myself in the mirror and try to smile like she was smiling in the picture, opening my mouth slightly and showing my top teeth. My face resists the upward curve of my lips. A smile looks out of place pressing on my filthy, tear-stained cheeks.

Setting the photograph on the vanity, I study my face in the mirror, running my fingers over it as if to reassure myself I'm really here. Thick black rings circle my eyes, and my skin has never looked so pale in the middle of summer before. My collarbone is protruding. It's been three days since I've eaten anything. Three days since I've given a shot. I touch my dry, peeling lips, and my fingernails catch my eye in the mirror. The polish has peeled off and my cuticles are cracking. The skin on my hands looks dehydrated, aging my wrinkled knuckles even more.

I feel the filth covering me. There are streaks of dirt across my face, and my hair is pressed flat against my head. When I scratch my neck, black grime collects under my nails. I step back and look down at my unshaven legs and bare feet. The dirt seems somehow symbolic. A sign of the struggle. I'm like a hungry artist who has endured the fast but still declines food. A shower is too easy.

Lowering myself onto the floor, I fold my head into my chest. I cry hard, harder than I've cried since I was a child. The tears turn to shouts, wails of rage, and I pound the side of the vanity with my fist to let it all escape. Every tear that falls and shout that escapes my lips makes me feel lighter. Finally, my body drained of energy, I curl into a ball on the cool tile floor. My eyes are swollen and my hair is soaked with tears. My lungs seem to spasm, trying desperately to smooth the flow of air moving in and out of the organs.

Finally, calm washes over me. My chest begins to rise and fall more slowly as my breathing evens out. I push myself up and curl my fingers around the side of the tub. With my knees pressed against the tile floor beneath me, I stare up at the showerhead. Kneeling like a praying child, I am fully exposed and vulnerable. I turn the hot water knob of the shower. Water gushes out as I peel my sweaty clothes off and step into the bathtub. I run handfuls of shampoo through my hair and pull the razor up my calves. Soap stings my already-burning eyes. I scrub every inch of my body until the water runs cold.

I remember a morning less than a month ago when Denise and I sprinted for the shower simultaneously. She broke into laughter as she gripped the shower curtain seconds before I did. The water heater is small, and the second shower of the morning inevitably ran cold. We both loved long, hot showers before breakfast. With a pair of clean underwear in my hand, I narrowed my eyes and stuck my tongue out at Denise. She raised her eyebrows in surprise and stuck her own tongue out back at me. I turned away from her and retreated to the kitchen.

The silly expression on my sister's face lingers in my mind as I step out of the shower and reach for my bathrobe on the back of the door. My hand stops in midair at the sight of Denise's terry cloth robe hanging next to mine. I take deep breaths as a lump forms in my throat. Sucking the steam from the shower into my lungs, I reach up and pull my own white robe from the hook. I feel comforted as I slide my arms into the sleeves and wrap the soft material around my body. I cover my dripping hair with a thick towel and step into the hall.

The Morgue

My sister's autopsy report finally comes in a large white envelope. I've been waiting for months. It's been lost in the stacks of paperwork at the county morgue and held up by the Department of Criminal Investigation. "It takes as long as it takes," the woman on the phone told me. And now the investigation is finally over. Hunched over my kitchen table, I light a cigarette and examine the envelope. Holding it up in one hand, I guess it contains about ten pages. I run my finger under the lip. My sister's full name greets me. Denise Irene Dominick. Her date of birth, date of death, and address. Former address. The cause of death has been ruled an accident. Coronary disease, a heart attack, the result of diabetes and cocaine abuse. As I flip through the pages, the details amaze me.

It states, "The body appears to be that of a well-developed, very thin, white female, consistent with the stated age of 33 years. The body is unclothed, cool to the touch, and preserved within normal limits. Measured height is 64 inches, scale weight is 90 lb. Rigor is absent. Scalp hair is brown, wavy, and 1 to 6 inches in length . . . The skin on the mid and lower abdomen shows prominent greenish discoloration . . . There is a 2 inch well-healed surgical scar oriented horizontally on the abdomen in the right lower quadrant. The external genitalia are those of a normal adult female. The legs are well-developed, symmetrical, and very thin . . . There are numerous healed needle puncture sites on the posterior and posterior lateral surfaces of the upper legs. The nails are clean and groomed very long . . . There is no unusual odor about the body."

I read it carefully. The report is inaccurate. She had bitten her nails to stubs her entire life. Her hair fell to the middle of her back. She'd been growing it out for months. It states her pancreas was healthy. My stomach drops as I stumble through the other details. There were holes in the lining of her nasal passages. Abscesses were detected on her lungs from smoking, and her liver had been damaged from too much alcohol throughout the years. I study the seemingly generic report with awe. It is too clinical, too formal, too bleak. The people who wrote it don't know her, but the words on these pages indicate that they know her thoroughly. She has become a case number.

The seasons changed while I waited for this report. The summer sun faded and crossed lower in the sky. Snow is on the ground outside this afternoon. Everything has moved forward, and the words on these pages hurl me back to that night that I guess I never really left behind. These pages are just a reminder. I thought that they would somehow bring closure, but the tightening in my chest that I haven't felt for months unexpectedly returns. I need an explanation.

I ENTER the county hospital through the automatic sliding doors and step up to the map encased in glass. My eyes scan the listings three times, but there is no sign of the morgue. I look around the lobby, expecting someone to ask me if I need directions. Men in ties rush by without looking my way, and a black woman in a wheelchair stares out the front window. This place is familiar only in that it's a hospital. Another hospital. Nothing more than that, I try to convince myself.

I stare down at my snow-covered shoes and contemplate a course of action. The medical examiner is expecting me. When I called to make an appointment, his secretary was indifferent. I told her I was a student, and she flatly told me to come the following Monday at one in the afternoon. Now I'm here, and nothing welcomes me.

Finally, I approach an efficient-looking man seated behind a large, wooden counter with the word INFORMATION across the front. I ask where the morgue is located. He gives me a sympathetic look, like I'm here to identify a body, and directs me to the basement.

A chill crawls up my back as I turn away from him. I'm not completely surprised at the underground location, but I haven't really prepared myself either. When I open the door to the stairs, I'm met by peeling yellow paint on the walls and cracked cement beneath my feet. The hallway is deserted and eerily silent. It smells wet. Goose bumps form on my arms like they would on a frightened child who has entered an abandoned house on a dare. I descend the flight of stairs slowly, pausing every few steps and looking back up toward the door to the lobby. My heels click on the cold floor. Finally, I reach a landing and push open the double doors marked COUNTY MORGUE.

The coroner doesn't meet me with a smile but rather frowns at the interruption. I recognize the deep lines on his pale face and the way his tired frame slumps slightly forward. His wire glasses rest on the end of his nose, and he studies me for several seconds. I gaze past him to the cluttered desk, politely letting him examine me. I remember his piercing blue eyes, but I know I'm not familiar to him. He has sat in many kitchens since he's been to my house several months ago. I don't expect him to know who I am. Like my sister during the autopsy, I am just another body.

He is strictly business as he walks ahead of me into the lab. He leans against a stainless steel counter and explains the autopsy procedure. The exterior of the body is examined first and then the usual Y-shaped incision is made to expose the internal organs. Body fluids are extracted by the pathologist. An autopsy is essentially dissecting a dead body. The procedure doesn't usually take more than two hours. Looking for anything out of the ordinary, they document identifying marks on the skin, weigh the organs, take tissue samples. Then they sew the body back up. There is satisfaction in the coroner's eyes when he tells me autopsies don't disfigure the bodies. "As good as new" are the words that come to my mind as I stand in front of a metal gurney.

Then he is silent. He's fulfilled his obligation to show a tax-payer and student around the facility. This is it, his eyes tell me. This is the room where it's all done. I search for my voice. I have questions.

"So you just do one at a time?" I ask.

The coroner smiles with a hint of pride and informs me that they have the accommodations to perform two autopsies at once.

"We've never done it though," he says.

"Never?" I ask, scribbling on the first page of my blank note-book.

"Well"—he pauses—"maybe once, but that was a long time ago and I'm sure it was just a freak occurrence. I think the pathologist that year was sick or we were behind schedule."

He reminds me that Des Moines does not have the homicide rate of some larger U.S. cities. The majority of Iowans die in accidents or from natural causes. Most of our bodies go from retirement homes or hospitals to the funeral homes in town. The medical examiner's scalpel will only touch a few of us. I follow him as he walks toward a metal door. It looks like a cooler in the kitchen of a restaurant.

"Oh, I remember," he continues, resting his hand on the metal latch and looking back at me. "It was the year our pathol-ogist had a heart attack. We just happened to have a couple cases come in on the same day. We ended up having to do them both at the same time."

"And then you send the people to the funeral home?" I ask. The word *people* sounds strange coming from my lips.

"Yes, as long as we can collect all the evidence we need. Sometimes we have to postpone a funeral a day or two. Not very often though," he replies.

The coroner opens the door and I see more stainless steel. There are no bodies in here, but there is space to comfortably fit eight adults. Shelves for the children. I look carefully around the large, walk-in freezer, squinting in the dim light, searching for blood. Then my eyes dart to the door. My sister's body was placed on an individual tray and closed behind the heavy stainless steel door. She was case number 93-0503 and her autopsy was performed at 9:09 A.M. I've memorized the details of the report.

"We can keep a body in here for several days. But the lab is pretty quick, and most of the time we find the cause of death relatively easily," he tells me.

A lump forms in my throat and my heart races as I imagine my sister's limp body resting on the cold metal hour after hour. The coroner senses my discomfort and motions around the cooler, talking about storage. I move slowly back into the examination room, maintaining eye contact with him as if I'm listening carefully to every word. Spots fill my eyes as my pupils try to adjust to the light in here. Lights everywhere, bouncing off the metal cupboards. Silver lamps stand upright in the corners and instruments are tucked away in drawers. The countertops sparkle too brightly, and the faint smell of formaldehyde lingers. Refrigerators hum as he talks about the procedure again.

"Pathologists always wear gloves when they're working," he says.

"AIDS?" I ask.

"We've become more concerned with the HIV virus in the past few years. It seems the virus continues to live in a dead body. The corpse becomes an incubator for diseases."

I nod, and he goes on to tell me that a white towel is sometimes placed over the head of the body during the autopsy.

I ask why.

"Personal choice," he replies. "Some pathologists just prefer not to see the . . . Well, they have a job to do here. Their primary concern is to find the cause of death, determine something that couldn't be determined at the scene or from medical records."

My sister didn't have any current medical records when she died. In her early twenties she just stopped going to doctors, never got physicals. I think she was afraid of doctors, feared what they would tell her. Sometimes, if she needed an antibiotic, she went to the county hospital. But she never told the nurses that she was a diabetic, because she said they would have treated her differently. She thought they would look for problems that she believed weren't there. She always told me that when you tell people you're diabetic, they immediately assume you're sick. I understood her fear of medical personnel and agreed with her theory about doctors being suspicious of my health. But as I stand in the basement of this hospital, I wish she would have trusted them more.

"So what if you don't find anything?" I ask, my words echoing between the walls.

"We always find something," he replies. There is unmistakable confidence in his voice. "It's not like *Quincy*."

I fake a smile and my eyes meet his. I'm suddenly filled with compassion for this man. I know the hardest part of his job is dealing with the living. He works with the dead for a reason.

Our conversation is interrupted when the outer door opens. I tell myself to look away, but my eyes are fixed on a man curled in the fetal position, being pushed through the doors on a gurney. I back up against a metal cupboard as two men in white shirts push him forward. They glance at me briefly before speaking to the coroner.

"A trucker. Found him out at Flying J's off the interstate. Looks like he's been dead several days," the taller man says. He pulls the arm away from the man's body and releases it. It is loose. "Rigor has already been here and gone."

Rigor mortis begins five to ten hours following death and disappears after two or three days. It helps the coroner determine a time of death. That man's muscles have stiffened and become loose again. The condition affects the muscles, and the body is held in the position it was in at the time of death. This explains why the man is curved like an unborn child. He was in that truck for too long. I can't pull my eyes away from him, thinking that someone should have found his body sooner. There is a wedding ring on his finger, and I wonder if a wife has been trying to contact him. The ring appears to be several sizes too small because his fingers have swelled.

"Identification?" the coroner asks.

"Yeah, we've got a name, but they haven't been able to locate any relatives yet. Looks like his home is in Nebraska and he was heading there. The back of the truck is empty. A waitress told us she thinks the truck has been sitting there for a few days." This man has an accent I can't place and stares at me as he speaks, wondering who I am and why I'm here.

And now I wish I weren't here because I recognize the bloating of the dead man's face. I know that enzymes and bacteria are decomposing him. The complex compounds of his skin and organs are being reduced to their components. He is becoming dust before my eyes. I know he hasn't always looked this way and hope that his wife doesn't ask to see him. He was probably very handsome before death went to work on him.

"He was slumped over the steering wheel." This is the first time the other man who wheeled the body in has spoken. He must be the driver.

"Probably a heart attack," the coroner says. He pulls a bottle of pills from the man's shirt pocket and reads the label. Then he slowly walks in a complete circle around the gurney, picking up the man's boot, checking his ears, lifting his eyelids. The coroner bends down and examines the dried blood under the man's nose.

"Go ahead and put him in." He motions toward the metal door. He has forgotten I'm here until he turns around to leave and sees me standing stiff-legged next to the counter.

"Well, you're welcome to come by in the morning and witness an autopsy firsthand if you'd like to," he tells me, exhaling loudly.

As I open my mouth to decline, I realize I'm not breathing.

I watch the driver pull the metal latch on the freezer as the other man pushes the gurney inside. They stay in the cooler for several minutes before returning with the empty stainless steel cart. As they push open the outer doors, I notice a note posted in the hall. It asks the medical personnel to be considerate of the hospital patrons. Make sure the double doors to the outer hallways are closed when delivering a body.

I can't help but envision a scalpel resting on my sister's bloated chest. I'd thought about the autopsy procedure before today, but the examination lights and metal bowls make the image chillingly real. I wonder if the towel completely covered her head. Just faceless hands working on her and a voice reporting the findings to a tape recorder. A surgery with no anesthesia. No fear of screwing anything up more than it already is. Denise's last contact with a doctor.

"Is it?" The coroner's voice catches my attention. He knows I haven't been listening.

"I'm sorry, what did you say?" I ask.

"Is this for a school report? Writing on the autopsy procedure?" he asks.

"Yes," I lie, wrapping my fingers around the copy of Denise's autopsy report in my pocket. "What are those for?" I ask, pointing to Polaroid photographs covering the wall outside the refrigerator door.

He replies that they remind the doctors what to look for. You learn from what you've seen before. I stare at the pictures.

Fragments of people jump out at me. A foot, a heart, a head wound. The burned foot is where the lightning bolt exited after striking a man. The heart in the photograph is covered with layers of white fat. A young man's head was torn apart by a bullet from a 9 mm. His hair is light brown. Pieces of people hang on the wall, and as I look at them I wonder if the coroner remembers any of the people behind the wounds.

The job here is too obvious. They deal in parts, not in whole people. I don't want to ask him the questions I thought I would about the autopsy findings. I suddenly don't need to know what it means when a peritoneum contains no blood or how the pathologist decompresses the neck organs to examine them. I don't want him to explain to me why my sister's pancreas was reported as being normal when she had diabetes. They said her eyes were blue. None of it matters anymore. I have no questions, because I know there are no answers here. My sister's soul doesn't dwell in this basement. I guess I knew bodies are only flesh, but the sterile instruments and the Polaroid photographs confirm it.

He glances at his watch, and I remove my hand from my jacket pocket, close the pad of paper my fingers were clenching.

"If you have the time and if you can be here by seven, you're welcome to come watch the autopsy in the morning. Premed students frequently come in and observe. It should be pretty quick. Coronary troubles are easier to diagnose," he tells me.

I shrug and look away to let him know I've seen enough. And then he cocks his head to the side, narrowing his eyes as though he might recognize me. I thank him for his time before he can speak.

I take the stairs two at a time. My lungs are aching as my foot bounces off the last step and I open the basement door. I rush through the lobby, through the automatic doors and outside. Live people pass me in the entryway. My feet hit the snow. Daylight envelops me and I inhale cold air deep into my lungs. I pull the pad of paper from my pocket and glance at the notes I've taken. Freezer. White towel. Eight adults. Always an explanation. I drop the pad of paper in a blue trash can near my car.

Decreased Visibility

I'M SITTING next to a stream near our camp when I first see the blood. My second day on this remote Alaskan trail. As I pump water through a filter and watch for salmon, everything I look at takes on a red tint. My right eye fills with bloody gel and black lines. I blink and rub my eye, but the vision won't clear. Time stops. My heart races and the muscles in my neck tense up. The water rushes by, drowning out all the other sounds of the wilderness and carrying all my energy downstream with it as I stare into the bloody mucus. The invincibility I felt hiking today drains from my numbing body. I run my hand over the rocky soil beneath me and wrap my fingers around my plastic coffee cup. Then I make my way back to the tent. I can see what looks like small, floating nerves. They're thin and bent like paper clips. Every time I move my eye, the debris gets disturbed and floats between me and the trees.

My friend Joel says it's probably just a retinal tear. He was making coffee when I asked him to look into my eye. He grabbed my shoulders and stared into the pupil, telling me to look in all directions. Then he shrugged and said he couldn't see anything. He told me the weight of the fifty-pound pack had just strained my body, that it could happen to anyone. He'd read about retinal tears. I could just as easily pull a hamstring or pop something out of joint. He told me I shouldn't worry, but I long to look at the eye myself. There are no mirrors here.

I've been in Alaska six weeks. Joel convinced me to take the trip with him, reminded me that life is short. We left in mid-May with a map, his dogs, and camping gear. I packed 200 syringes and four vials of insulin in the bottom of my pack. Enough to last if I reuse the needles. As Joel backed down my driveway the morning of our departure, I slipped my sunglasses over my eyes and propped my feet on the cracked dash. The dogs paced the length of the truck box, and smoke from Joel's Marlboro drifted through the cab. Energized by a sense of adventure, I rolled my window down and turned up the stereo.

South Dakota met us with light rain, and Montana with the first stirrings of spring. Pitching our tent in the early evening, we prepared dinner over our propane burner and built a fire as the sun set through the trees. The Rocky Mountains loomed before us, overtaking the sky. We stopped for moose that loped lazily across the highway and deer that darted in front of our truck. I soaked up the landscape each day, endlessly amazed at the picture-perfect beauty of the Northwest. Clouds hung like halos around the tops of the snowcapped mountains. Evergreens climbed for miles over rolling hills.

Some days we would drive 300 miles and others only 50. We kept no schedule and spent three days soaking in natural hot springs in Canada. I read books about the forests and trails I would meet in Alaska, took pictures, wrote letters to friends at home, and scribbled in my journal. We met people from all around the country and shared stories of our home states over campfires late into the night. Joel and I ate breakfast in roadside cafes and hiked trails with the dogs in the afternoon. My memories of home seemed like they should belong to someone else.

The trip up the Alaska Highway was hard. We drove for hours every day on gravel, waiting while construction trucks repaired the heavily traveled roads in front of us. The roar of machinery interrupted the silence. Joel and I started to argue about where to pitch the tent or what to listen to on the radio. A friendship growing tense from the stress. Washing in a stream went from being a pleasure to being a nuisance. Campgrounds were packed with RVs and logging trucks forced us onto the shoulder of the highway. The tedious driving put a strain on us, but when we finally arrived in the heart of Alaska, our passion returned. It was breathtaking.

Open sky and untouched wilderness humbled me. The vast, traversed trails were intimidating, but I craved conquering them. We hiked overgrown paths that drained me physically. My feet hurt and the pack became heavy as we climbed steep paths through Wrangell–St. Elias. Some days my body seemed too tired to continue, and my blood sugar would plummet from overexertion. I sucked on candy to keep moving and fell asleep before I could get my boots off at the end of the day. Viewing the landscape firsthand had its price in the form of blisters and lower-back aches, but it was worth it. I was filled with pride every time I made it to the top of a summit or the end of a trail.

But now my eye is presenting a different sort of challenge. I look around the tent, wishing I could enjoy the solitude I had sought so eagerly only two months ago. Instead, I long for a doctor or hospital. I'm scared. As much as I dream about finding peace out here in isolation, the reality is that I will always need civilization. I will always need medical supplies. As rain starts to fall softly outside, I ache for something comfortable. Closing my eyes tightly, I wish the blood away.

The mosquitoes will be out soon. Sheep Camp, the second stop on this trail, is starting to fill up with other hikers who plan to attempt the pass tomorrow. The rangers told us to allow ten hours to make the steep climb over the summit. It had been labeled the "Golden Stairs" because it involves an elevation gain of 1,000 feet in less than half a mile. A 45-degree angle of rocks and snow. And if it isn't clear, if visibility is reduced, we were told, we shouldn't attempt it. I think of the irony of this advice as I blink my eyes again. I can only see bits and pieces of objects through my right eye, but we've already hiked fifteen miles in the footsteps of the stampeders to get to the base. I'm tired, but I can't stop.

I wonder about those who have gone before us on this trail. Those seeking gold. The Chilkoot Trail had been used by the Chilkoot Indians as a trade route before the white man discovered it in the late 1800s. It was a shorter but more arduous route to the mines. Single families carried all their possessions, hundreds of pounds, over this terrain. They were looking for a better life, and I guess that's what I'm doing here too. Something better. New. Denise has been dead for a year, and I'm moving on with my life. When I return I'll be entering my first semester of graduate school, but I needed to come here first.

Stretching out on my back, I reflect on the last few days. Yesterday, four hours onto this trail, I knew this was going to be the most difficult thing I'd ever done. I hoped my body wouldn't fail me. My feet hurt and the pack felt heavy, but only because I was thinking about it. I learned to lose myself in my thoughts as my legs pumped. Instead of concentrating on my muscles, I became pensive. Removed myself from the physical. And when I became aware of the strain again, I reminded myself that I had chosen to be here, had dreamed about being in Alaska.

It's just that my dreams didn't include the debris in my eye. I know a little bit about diabetic retinopathy, and I know seeing blood is a symptom. I wish I could believe what Joel says about a retinal tear, but memories of half-heard doctors' advice haunt me. Diabetes is the leading cause of adult blindness. My sister always said she'd kill herself if she went blind. She didn't want to live if she couldn't experience the world through her eyes. She argued that listening and touching wouldn't be enough for her, but she never had any problems with her vision. I try to convince myself that I'm as lucky, try to forget what I know about how the disease slowly wears on the blood vessels in my body. The mosquitoes begin to buzz outside the tent.

Our cheap tent. Other hikers have more expensive ones. We

got ours at a department store back in Des Moines. It's light for packing, but it isn't standing up to the conditions like we'd hoped it would. Even though Joel rain-proofed it, condensation is slowly accumulating inside. The thin material barely separates me from the elements. Joel says the best thing about being out here in the middle of nowhere is that we will realize how fragile we really are. He thinks it's important to separate ourselves from the comforts of civilization to realize we're human, and he says we have to challenge our mortality to really live. I just wonder how far my limits can be pushed. The body is never as strong as the spirit that drives it. My stomach rumbles and I know I have to eat something. I'll have to go outside among the other hikers because a bear was spotted in this camp last night, and Joel has strict rules about not eating in the tent. But I realize I've lost my fear of bears now, as if I know that animal will not be the thing to take my life.

Pulling my boots behind me, I crawl out of the tent. Hikers have gathered near a small Forest Service cabin. There are probably twenty-five men and women cooking on propane stoves, eating candy bars, and laughing. Their voices reflect both fatigue and excitement as they anticipate the upcoming trip over the pass. When bad weather slowed the gold-seekers in the late 1800s, 3,000 to 6,000 people could be found in Sheep Camp at any one time. We are still below tree line here and sheltered from some of the rain. Joel is stirring something in a pan and smiles when he sees me.

"It's about time you got up," he laughs.

I look past him to his backpack and ask if we have any cheese left. He tells me it's wrapped in plastic in the stream to keep it cold. Grabbing a knife from the food bag, I head toward the water. He turns down the flame on the small burner and follows me.

"What's wrong? Worried about the pass tomorrow?" he asks.

"Not really. A little nervous, but not scared."

"It can't be as tough as they say," he replies. "Don't worry."

I want to tell him I can barely see out of my right eye. It's getting worse. The blood is still there, but what looks like a thick, cloudy gel has accumulated. I want to describe to him what I'm seeing, but I'm afraid to say anything out loud. It will make it too real.

So I slice cheese with a rust-stained knife while we talk about the trail. Spending day after day together, our discussions are now focused on the immediate. During our drive up, we exhausted philosophical and rhetorical conversations. In the cab of the truck, we had told all the stories of our pasts and hopes for our futures. Now the conversations revolve around what we do each day. We exist in the moment, no longer acknowledging who we had been or what we had done before we arrived in Alaska.

The summit is in full view from where we are. It looks like a mountain of snow. The rain has let up and the sun is making its way out from behind a cloud. I've finally adjusted to the twenty-some hours of sunlight each day. I try to stare into the sun, as if it has the power to burn through the haze of blood.

"Lots of people showing up," Joel remarks.

"Have you talked to any of them?" I ask, pulling my eyes from the sky and nodding toward a group of tents.

"Yeah, a few. Most are Canadians. That guy over there is from Germany," Joel says, pointing his fork at a young blond man stirring something in a pan over his stove. "Looks pretty cute, huh?"

I nod. Normally, I listen carefully to Joel, picking out the little bits of humor in his words. But today I am barely hearing him. I seem to exist completely outside our conversation. My mind has surrendered complete, undivided attention to my eye.

The German looks over at us and Joel waves. The man raises his hand in return. Bound to us by common experience.

"So," Joel continues, "are you missing home yet?"

"No." I pause before continuing. "I wouldn't mind a hot

bath right now or a dry place to sleep, but I don't miss it." My words sound convincing and Joel winks at me.

"I told you you'd love it," he says. "Sometimes when I start thinking I'd like to go home, I remember the feeling I got driving through the city traffic every afternoon. The stress. The mere presence of other drivers elevated my blood pressure. So, it was sign up for a yoga class or come to Alaska. All I have to do is imagine myself in my truck on a backed-up freeway at eight in the morning, and I'm overwhelmed to fall to my knees and thank God that I'm here." He does fall to his knees, but instead of prayer, he kisses the damp earth and laughs.

Smiling down at the top of his head, I can understand his love for this place. The peace I have found here in the wilderness is like none I have ever experienced. I will never be able to explain to the people back home the serenity of the wind in the trees or the unity I feel with nature. Our friends couldn't understand why we wanted to come here. They said they didn't know what was fun about spending the summer without showers or television. They asked what we were running from. Or running to. My mother thought I was crazy. She had watched a television show on bear attacks and didn't want me to go, but I replied that there are risks to our lives everywhere. I had a greater chance of getting shot in downtown Des Moines than I did being mauled by a bear in Alaska. She said that at least she'd know I was dead if I got shot in Des Moines. She'd still have a body to bury. Next to her other daughter's. I walked out of the house that day and slammed the door.

My dad had looked worried but wished me well. He knew this was more than just a vacation for me. He understood that it was something I had to do. He told me that if he were twenty-three years old with no attachments, he would probably head up to Alaska himself, but I knew that he would miss me. We spent a lot of time together after Denise died, riding our bikes and meeting for coffee after the late news. The day I left for Alaska, he handed me a phone card, an envelope full of ten-dollar bills, and a pair of binoculars.

"My parents are probably worried sick," I say quietly. "We haven't called in over a week."

Joel doesn't hear me because he's watching the German. I study my hiking partner's profile. A strong jaw. The stubble on his face makes him look rugged and seems out of character. He's too soft-spoken to look so tattered. We've been friends for almost four years and I thought I knew him well, but we seem to be changing this summer. Both finding and losing our true selves out here.

We walk back to the rock where Joel had been preparing his food. I follow his gaze to the German. Perched on a fallen tree, he shovels noodles into his mouth straight from the pan with a plastic fork.

"He looks like a lumberjack," I comment to Joel.

"Huh?" he asks. "Yeah, well . . ." His voice trails off and he concentrates on the meal he's preparing.

"Want some of this?" he asks, holding up the pan.

I look inside. Beef stew from a package. None of the vegetables have soaked up any of the water and they are floating around on top, separated from the brownish broth beneath them. I shake my head slowly from side to side.

Though my stomach growls, I've lost any desire to eat. Sleep is what I long for. Close my eyes and wake up with clear vision. But I know I'll lie awake all night, listening to the sounds of the forest and the snores of the other campers. I will stare at the walls of the tent and worry about my eye.

"Do you?" I hear Joel's voice.

"What?" I ask.

"Do you want to go with me to talk to the German?"

I shake my head and run my fingers through my hair. The grease feels slippery on my skin.

"I'm going to go wash up," I tell him. He shrugs, grabs a handful of trail mix, and turns his thin back to me. His rain jacket is torn and mud looks permanently caked to his hiking boots. I look down at my soiled sweatshirt, feeling ashamed of the filth for the first time since I've been in Alaska. Rummaging through Joel's pack, my fingers find the biodegradable soap, and I head to the water.

Sitting on the bank of the rushing stream, I look up to the summit again. It dares me to climb, challenges me to beat it. I've never seen anything so beautiful. My eyes follow it slowly from the base to the peak, and I know I'll find the energy to make my way up. Denise would tell me it's all mental. The image of my sister's rounded, laughing face fills my head. She told me once that people can muster inhuman strength from the mind. Strength we couldn't imagine we possessed. But she'd never seen this mountain. I wonder if she is laughing at me. Stuck in the middle of nowhere with a backpack full of dehydrated food and an eye full of blood. If she were here, she would tell me I'd gotten myself into quite a situation. Then she'd laugh and tell me how to get myself out of it. Which would probably be just to keep moving up the path.

I dip my head into the icy stream. I can't be far from the source of the water, probably a glacier somewhere on the top of the mountain. My scalp goes numb as I try to lather the soap in my hair, wishing that I had never started washing it. The cold makes my head ache even more. Looking down and trying to get a clear image of myself in the water, I strain to see the details of my face, catch a glimpse of my eye. But the water flows too quickly and I can't make out anything, so I just dip my head into the water. Biting my lip, I hold back a cry as the freezing flow catches my hair. Finally, I stand up and let the icy drops fall into the stream.

I head to the tent and arrange my belongings around me on my sleeping bag. Deet, pepper spray, a small bottle of unscented hand lotion, insulin and needles, a bottle of filtered water. And I close my eyes. Because it is the only way I can escape the blood. It starts to rain again, and I listen to the sound of the drops falling through the leaves of the trees onto the tent. I stretch my neck and hold my head outside. With my face to a sky I can't see, tears well beneath my eyelids. I am fully aware of the solitude I have come here to find.

Pamphlets

THE DOCTOR IS telling me she will insert a needle into the lower part of my eye socket and immobilize the muscles in the eye. I stare at the white walls while she explains the procedure and hands me a pastel pamphlet giving me the statistics on diabetic retinopathy. It tells me I'm not alone but also makes me realize I'm not one of the fortunate ones who detected their condition early.

My eyes dilated, I turn the pamphlet over in my hands, barely seeing the print. I almost laugh at the irony. I wonder if there is a closet somewhere in the back of the office used only for the storage of pamphlets. In the waiting room, I looked around and noticed that every patient seemed to be holding a green, pink, or light blue pamphlet. Different colors for different conditions. And I guess there is some comfort in having one to take home. It's as if they know you will remember nothing they have said. They send you away with a reminder, something tangible. This pamphlet has a picture of the inner eye. An eye that's not functioning properly.

I feel better in knowing someone went to the trouble to write it all down. I think if there's a pamphlet about it, it can't be that rare. I calculate in my head that approximately 80 percent of diabetics who have had the disease fifteen years or longer develop some degree of retinopathy. I should not be surprised to find myself in this office, because I've gone fourteen years without complications. Maybe I should feel fortunate somehow. As if I'm normal.

The room is all white, and I squint to see the framed university diplomas on the wall, but I can't make out any of the writing. Next to a degree from the University of Iowa there is a huge diagram of a retina. A healthy eye. None of the blood vessels are leaking. A large piece of equipment stands between the doctor and me. Just minutes before, she used it on my eyes in order to see the blood vessels that have weakened and hemorrhaged. She gazed at them a long time, and it was during those minutes I knew there was a more serious problem than I had first anticipated.

I've been home from Alaska two days, and I asked my father to bring me to this office today. I had held some hope that it was going to be a retinal tear, but this pamphlet in my hand says "Diabetic Retinopathy" in large white letters. I've read the books on diabetes and I know that lack of oxygen has caused the vessels in the back of my eye to weaken. Fifteen years of Type I diabetes can have this effect. A few vessels have already broken and caused some vision loss in my right eye. The debris from the hemorrhage is floating around back there, preventing light from hitting my retina. I will have to undergo laser surgeries to prevent more vessels from bursting.

The doctor gets my attention by tapping on the pamphlet in my hand with her pencil. She knows I have not been listening because she sees ten of my kind every day. She gives me that knowing look, as if I am going to be one of the difficult ones, the young woman who leaves today and then returns with a list of written questions next week, so she continues to talk about what she knows. Procedures.

"And about that injection into your cheek . . . ," she begins again.

She says this nonchalantly as if another needle shouldn't be a problem for a diabetic. Doctors frequently do this. They believe I have no fear of needles. Perhaps they are about to tell me it will pinch for a second before remembering who I am. Then they say nothing. They do this with booster shots, Novocain, and even when they're drawing blood from a vein. I know this woman will probably do the same thing when I go in for surgery next week. She will remember that this is diabetic retinopathy. That I am a diabetic. And she will give me no reassuring words before insertion but will be frighteningly silent, even though she has a lot to say right now.

"You'll need to notify your primary physician. Do you have a physician?" she asks.

I simply stare at her and nod my head, knowing I will not report this to Dr. Manning. He will be too concerned. He will make a big deal out of it and insist on blood tests and kidney checks. He'll want to search for other diabetic complications. He has watched me grow up, and now I don't want to tell him about this eye problem. I don't want him to think I haven't taken care of myself.

"Who is your doctor?" the woman before me asks.

When I tell her, she raises her eyebrows and suggests I find another doctor, one who specializes in diabetes. I need to monitor my blood sugars more closely. High blood sugars are probably what led to the weakening and breaking of these vessels in the first place, she says. She is telling me things I know. She writes down the names of some doctors and hands me the paper. I stare at her immaculate fingernails and tuck the little list of faceless names inside the pamphlet. It's as if she believes these people will save my sight, save my life. She assumes I have faith in doctors.

And to a certain degree I do. I have to. I need to trust this woman, because she called my case severe. I wonder what she sees when she looks through that lens into my eyes. I have no choice but to trust her. This isn't a lesion on my skin or a pain in my gut she is talking about. This isn't something I can look in the mirror and see. The breaks are behind the lens of my eye, and no one can see them but her. I glance at the diplomas on the wall again.

"We do several of these surgeries every week," she reassures me. "You are a bit young to have developed this condition, but we've seen younger."

And I was, by far, the youngest person in the waiting room here. Most of my friends just go to optometrists where they read the eye chart and get their new glasses. The people in the waiting room of this office had eyes sixty or seventy years old. I think one can reasonably expect some problems by then. But there was one small child who came out of the back room. A nurse was leading her by the hand. With a white patch covering her left eye, the child stretched her free hand in front of her, feeling her way through the air toward her parents. The little girl's mother was holding a pamphlet and brushing away tears as she rose to put her arms around her daughter. When the girl finally focused on her mom and saw the tears, she started crying herself. I watched them together, stared at the child's tanned legs and scraped-up knees, wondered how long it would be before she played outside again. Wondered if she was going blind, because she couldn't have been more than four or five years old.

Waiting rooms always make my skin clammy, but I wish I could go back in time thirty minutes and stare at the overstuffed magazine racks out there. Thirty minutes ago my life wasn't being shattered. Phil Donahue's lips moved on the silent television screen, and I studied the faces of the people around me. They watched as the office door opened and closed. They waited. They waited for spouses undergoing exams and surgeries, waited for the results of tests, waited while their pupils dilated, waited for their own names to be called. Waiting rooms possess a mood of their own. Tension and relief all hang in the air simultaneously. Nervous sighs escape some visitors as they glance at their watches, while others are perfectly content to remain in the plastic chairs for hours. My father is waiting for me there.

". . . and then you'll have to wear a patch for a while," the doctor continues.

She tells me about the gauze patch required after the surgery. It keeps the light out of the eye, and I can take it off after eight hours. There will be a little bruise under my eye where the needle was inserted. After I take the patch off, I will have to put drops in my eye for three days to keep the pupil dilated and the muscles relaxed. My vision will be blurred, and I will feel like someone punched me. The trauma to the eye from the laser surgery will also cause me to see spots for several days and I will lose some night vision.

She is going to cauterize the outermost blood vessels my eye uses to see when the pupil is dilated. And then I will have the vision of the old. I've heard their complaints about the way they can't see the lines on the road at night and how the headlights of other drivers make visibility hard. I will learn how to drive again.

Seeing in a dimmed room will be more difficult after the surgeries. I will buy another lamp for my living room and use brighter lightbulbs after the surgery. I will learn to use my hands to find objects in the dark, and my sense of touch will become more keen. I will rely on my fingertips to find the keys in the bottom of my purse or to open my car door at night. Vision loss is a result of this treatment. This doctor tells me it's inevitable.

Inevitability will become interchangeable with destiny. I will try to learn to accept the fact that my fate is in the hands of the doctors. Never having asked for help before, I will be forced to rely on them to stabilize the condition. I will learn to ask. I will tell Ann that I can't drive at night. She will maneuver her car across the busy streets of Des Moines and come ten miles out of her way to pick me up. I will learn to swallow my pride, pick up the telephone, and dial the telephone numbers of my friends. I will hear a familiar voice and then the sound of my own voice. Asking for help.

"You shouldn't lift anything over ten pounds either. No running. Don't do anything rigorous," she continues.

"For how long?" I ask.

"We're not sure. We only know that sudden increases in blood pressure or simple physical strain can cause vessels to unexpectedly break."

I wonder who the *we* is she is referring to. Doctors always talk like this. As if when one speaks, they all speak. I think of the Borg character on *Star Trek*. The collective. Every brain is connected to one big database, and no independent thought is permitted.

But this doctor is human, and I struggle to remember that. She probably has children and a dog at home. Maybe even has medical problems of her own. I don't know about her life, though I find myself longing to know something about her. Something other than what I see before me. White coat. Brown hair pulled away from her round face. Manicured nails wrapped around a clipboard. Moving easily around my chair, she feels at home within this white room. I want to know what she does when she leaves her office at night, but she continues to talk about what the surgery will be like. And when she notices that I am not listening, she sighs. The sigh a parent gives to a small child. A sigh that she gives to my kind every day. I find some comfort in that, as I do in the pamphlet.

So I let that woman with perfect nails perform four surgeries, two on each eye, over the course of the next two months. Just before the fourth surgery, I am sitting on the hospital bed, waiting for her to arrive, and I pick up my medical chart. She has written the words "severe, high-risk, proliferative diabetic retinopathy" on the top of one of the pages. The words scare me. She walks in while I'm reading and takes the folder from my hand, as if I haven't the right nor the knowledge to understand its contents. I never return to her after that day. I decide I'm not going to go anywhere else either. I read a medical book on diabetic retinopathy and discover that two surgeries are usually sufficient. But a week later another vessel breaks.

I'm leaning over to turn on my television when I see the familiar blood and debris behind my left eye. I watch the vessel break and bleed and block my vision as I listen to the weather report. I can see the tiny nerves scattering behind my lens, so I close my eyes. I sit on my living room floor and listen to the broadcast about the killings in the Middle East. The reporter is referring to pictures on the screen, but I keep my eyes closed. I think about having to go back to that woman. With vision in only one eye, I dial information and get the phone number for the University of Iowa Hospital. I read in a magazine that their ophthalmology department ranks in the top five in the nation. I hope for a more compassionate doctor. One who would tell me that the insertion of that needle is going to pinch for a second.

THIS DOCTOR tells me to stare at a spot on the ceiling. I have to keep my eyes open as he inserts the needle into my eye socket. I shift my gaze from the ceiling to his eyes as he pushes down the plunger, and I feel the burning solution enter my muscle. I stare at him standing above me, trying to cling to the image of his sympathetic hazel eyes as everything goes dark. The left side of my face goes numb. When I reach up to touch my own cheek, it's as though I am no longer a physical presence in this room, unable to feel my own fingertips resting on my face, unable to see my own hand. The doctor leads me through a door marked DANGER—RADIATION, and I sit down behind the familiar machine and rest my chin on the towel. Laser lights fill my eyes. I count the blasts to keep my mind occupied. Tears stream down my face. I'm not in pain, just tired.

The drive to get to the University of Iowa Hospital was long. My father and I left Des Moines last night, but the interstate was closed about thirty miles east of the city due to the weather. Blinding snow enveloped our car, and my father couldn't see.

He leaned toward the windshield and opened his eyes wide, trying to catch a glimpse of other cars we knew were somewhere ahead of us. I stared through the windows into pure white.

Luckily we found a hotel room along the road, but we got no sleep. I could sense my father's nervousness the entire night. As if he should have had control over the snowstorm or was failing to get his daughter help. I told him not to worry, that both the blinding snow and the debris in my eye were beyond his control. I said that the blood was already beginning to settle out of my eye. I sat on the double bed next to him and pretended to read a magazine, even though I could barely make out the photographs of the models in the advertisements.

All night my father kept reaching over and patting my hand, asking me if I needed anything. Normally I would have found humor in a gesture like that, considering it was so obvious there was nothing he could do. We were stuck in a hotel full of college kids trying to get home for the weekend and businessmen missing their wives, and I had an eyeful of blood. Finally, my father leaned back against the headboard and pushed buttons on the remote control, staring at the wall above the television.

Today the doctor is doing what he referred to as "heavy laser" on my left eye. He explained that after this surgery I will probably notice the most significant loss of vision yet. There are still hundreds of weak vessels back there, vessels that if left untreated will explode. If more and more break, the fluid might accumulate behind my retina and cause it to detach. He said then we'd have an even bigger problem on our hands. So he's using a laser to force the weak vessels to regress. Then it takes several weeks to know whether or not the eye has responded to the surgery. He said it can sometimes take up to two years for this condition to stabilize in someone my age. They say a person over sixty might need fewer surgeries, whereas someone in their twenties could require more. Younger bodies try to heal themselves by attempting to regenerate the vessels the doctors force into regression.

"You're not going to go blind," he says, as if reading my mind. I've counted to 500. "You've lost some peripheral vision, night vision, and things will be dimmer, but you're not going blind right now."

I say nothing. I think about my sister, wondering what she would do if she were the one sitting in this room. Denise always told me people didn't have to know that we were diabetic and having the disease wouldn't change my life. But now it has. My life is different. Not just because I can barely see to drive at night or because my father is reading entire novels to me. My life has changed because I am finally facing who I am. Who I have become. I was always in complete control of my life, and now I have to accept sacrificing this control to other people. I need their help and I'm learning to face this reality. I have to try to believe the doctor's words and have faith in them as I would a religious scripture. And in three months, this is the first time anyone has told me that I wasn't going completely blind right now. I had been afraid to ask. Scared to say the word *blind* out loud and afraid of what they would tell me. But this doctor said the words. *You're not going blind right now.*

It could happen in the upcoming years from glaucoma or macular degeneration or retinal detachment, but not right now. Not from this condition. I will remember this doctor's words in the upcoming months. When my eyes don't respond to these laser treatments, while I wait for those little vessels to shrivel up and die, I will accept my condition. My vision will get worse, but I'll adjust to it. Eventually it won't seem like I'm waiting to go blind or waiting to die as much as I'm learning how to see the world more clearly. I will simultaneously lose and gain my vision.

The next time I'm in this hospital, the doctors will tell me that the vessels aren't responding to the surgeries as they'd hoped they would. They'll say that some people go through several laser treatments and there still isn't any improvement. The doctors will stand in the examining room with me, holding photographs of my retina, and discuss a course of action. But my heart won't race anymore in their presence. When the vessels in my eye refuse to shrivel up and die from their treatments, refuse to be burned and shrink up, and continue to grow and break, I'll embrace their will to survive. Their desire to grow in response to the doctors' attempts to kill them. A few months from now, when the doctors line up the pictures of my retina before me, side by side, and talk about risks and options, I won't tense up. I'll sit back in the chair and close my eyes and breathe. Because I'll believe in my life, the life my body is fighting for.

Right now, my back tight and neck cramped, I hold my breath and count the laser bursts, feeling the rays of light like little fires inside my head, thinking for a moment about radiation and cancer. When my count reaches 735, the doctor pulls me away from the machine. He pats my shoulder and talks about the advancements that have been made in treating diabetics. I feel safe with this man.

I saw the diplomas on his office wall. His wife is expecting their second child. They've been married for six years, and the wedding band on his finger is too tight for his chubby hand. His hair is thinning and his glasses are scratched and he knows about diabetes. He had talked to me for a long time before he inserted that needle into my cheek. He even let me see my medical file when I asked and explained to me what the jargon meant.

"How is it, then, that diabetics so often go blind?" I ask.

He sighs. But it is a thoughtful sigh. He tells me that it is mainly people who do not seek care.

"They ignore the blood they see in their eyes," he says. "They assume it will go away and things will just heal up if they leave it alone. Sometimes by the time they get here they can't see anything through all the debris behind the lens. And we have to wait to do surgeries because we can't see anything either. Other people don't even know they have diabetes, but there are some diabetic eye conditions we can't do anything for at this time. However, you're so young . . ."

I can barely see him, but I nod because I know there is compassion in his eyes.

". . . and we're seeing more and more young people like yourself with this condition," he continues. "Individuals who developed diabetes as children and ran high blood sugars through their adolescent years. They tend to think themselves invincible. They don't listen to medical advice."

I understand what he is telling me, and he knows it. He pats my shoulder, smooths back my hair, and tapes a gauze patch over my eye.

"Do you have any other questions?" he asks.

I shake my head. The questions I have are not ones he can answer.

He breathes deeply and settles back into his chair. "You have to be sure you're testing your blood sugars every day, Andie," he says.

"I am," I reply.

"And going to the doctor for blood work," he continues.

I nod. Last month I went to see Dr. Manning and asked him about new diabetic medications to help control blood sugars. He had narrowed his eyes and asked me if I was having some kind of problem. I lied that everything was fine and told him that I had just decided it was time for me to really start being more careful. He prescribed a new drug called Metformin. It was supposed to aid in the utilization of insulin, but it made me sick. And my blood sugars weren't any lower. It only works if your pancreas is still secreting some insulin, and mine has been completely dead for many years. It helps some Type II diabetics, but he told me I could try it out for a little while and see if it made any difference. I stayed on it for three weeks, throwing up every morning. I stopped taking it, but I just read yesterday about a new medication that should be approved by the FDA this month. It's supposed to slow the absorption of carbohydrates and keep the blood sugar from elevating so quickly. I'm going to go back to Dr. Manning and ask him about that one next week.

"I am being careful," I repeat to this doctor sitting before me.

"Good," he replies. "You have to think about your kidneys. Your eye problems are a sign that the disease has harmed the blood vessels in your body. That means the nerves in your feet, legs, and some internal organs might not be getting the oxygen they need either." He takes a deep breath. "And you've had the disease for several years. You've got to think more than you probably want to about where you're going to be in five or ten years."

My head is starting to ache, and I don't feel like talking about the future right now. I start to stand up and he takes my arm, leads me back to the waiting room where my father is reading a magazine. With the Valium weighing on me, I will sleep while my father drives 100 miles back to Des Moines through this December blizzard.

My dad walks me down the hall to the elevator. I can see out of my right eye, but that too is blurry from broken vessels and repeat surgeries over the past few months. I'm not paying attention and I run into a medical cart. Something falls, but my father says nothing, grasps my arm more firmly, and maneuvers me around it.

When we get outside, the sun is blinding. My dad eases me onto a bench and I wait in the cold while he goes to get the car. I keep my eyes closed, but I can feel people walk by. I assume they are staring. Wondering to themselves what could be wrong with the eyes of such a young woman. A man pauses in front of me. I can smell his cologne and he asks in a sympathetic voice if I need help getting somewhere. Holding my chin to my chest, fumbling for my sunglasses in my purse, I tell him thanks anyway. I can hear him hesitating as he walks away. Others continue to pass by, but I am sure I only hold their attention for a moment. They, too, are carrying pamphlets in their pockets. Detached retinas, macular degeneration, cornea transplants, AIDS-related eye complications. I am not alone as I feel the familiar grasp of my father's hand.

Alone

I PULL BACK THE creaking doors on the shed and look inside at the clutter. Several boxes labeled with black felt markers are stacked high against the back wall. My sister's things. A rusting, broken lawn mower holds three folding chairs in place against the boxes. Pushing gardening tools aside with my foot, I lean forward and move my hiking gear out of the way before grabbing my mountain bike. Crumpled leaves are still stuck in the spokes from last fall. I wheeled this hefty bike in here when the first snow flew. I was rushing to get plastic on the windows that day. It has been a long winter.

One snowstorm after another swept through the Midwest, and just when I thought spring was about to arrive, the temperature would plummet and more snow would fall. Driving was difficult for me. If it was snowing lightly, I could usually make it to my destination, but if the flakes started to come down more quickly, I'd grip the steering wheel tightly and leaned forward toward the windshield. Visibility was worse at dusk, and I tried to avoid driving at night altogether. Some afternoons I would step out of my car and find my whole body had cramped up from all the stress of driving in the falling snow. I longed for this spring and the sunshine to finally arrive.

My cocker spaniel tilts his head to the side and watches me. Holly and I found Sidney eight months ago at the animal shelter. He was sitting alone in a cage in the corner, shivering from fear, terrified of everyone who approached his cage. A big sign that read I'M SIDNEY—PLEASE TAKE ME HOME was fastened to the wire. I walked right past him, but Holly stopped. Her long blond hair fell around her face as she kneeled down and spoke softly to him, repeating his name over and over. Then she reached up and opened the door. Sidney didn't move. I looked down the cement corridor, waiting for an attendant to appear and yell at Holly to put the dog back in. She cradled him in her arms and said that he was the one for me. I replied that he was too small and moved on to a cage with two German shepherd puppies. "Look, they're brothers," I told her. She ignored the other dogs and followed me with Sidney in her arms, told me I'd be sorry if I didn't adopt him.

Then a guy appeared behind her. I waited for the reprimand. But when he circled around her, he looked rushed and suburban. Not an employee. "Ya gonna buy this dog?" he asked, rubbing Sidney's long ear between his thumb and index finger. She immediately answered yes. Lied that the adoption proceedings were already in the process. We were taking him home. I couldn't believe what I was seeing. It was like a used car lot and the agency had sent this decoy out to pressure us. I rolled my eyes and turned away. Holly adopted the dog and left him at my house that afternoon. Now I can't remember what my life was like before I had him. He sleeps next to me on the bed at night, and slams his paw into the metal bowls when I forget to feed him. He goes everywhere with me, but today I'm going to ride alone.

Walking my bike down the driveway, I study my neighbors' houses. Boxy and boring. They all have shutters. The lawns are trimmed and garbage cans are stacked neatly against the garages. I've thought about moving several times since Denise died. I had a roommate for a while. Michele slept in Denise's old bedroom, and we talked over coffee in the kitchen late into the night. But eventually we needed our own space. I prefer living alone, living with Sidney. And I can't move from this house.

I don't know any of my neighbors very well. My sister used to talk to them, but I keep to myself. The mailbox at the end of the driveway next door reads "Hutchins." They have three kids, and sometimes I wave when they pull up in their minivan. Dave lives on the other side of me. He has a girlfriend, and I've lost track of the kids who visit. Products from previous marriages. After Denise died, I felt uncomfortable around the neighbors, like a freak. They all have families. I have no children who can play with theirs, and I never turn on my porch light on Halloween.

Stopping at the end of my driveway to pump up my bike tire, I spot a man across the street getting out of his car. I've noticed him before, but we've never spoken. He looks about my age, and I watch as he sets his briefcase down on the hood of his car and opens the passenger's side door. I tilt my head to the side and pretend to be preoccupied with my tire. Through the blue frame of my bike, I watch as he pulls tools from his trunk. He's tall with light hair and his movements are smooth. I look at my watch. 10:30. The pavement warms beneath me, and I stand up.

With open road ahead of me, I push the red button on my odometer. I know where I'm headed. The water. The stream I have spent hours sitting by. I'll check to see if my lawn chair has survived the winter. I tucked it under the railroad bridge last fall, knowing it would be months before I stretched out on it again. Last summer after I returned from Alaska, I went there alone every Saturday. I pretended I was still up north and watched the shallow water run over my feet, looking for the salmon I'd never see in Iowa. After learning about my eye problems, I kept to myself most of the time. Thinking. No one else ever goes to the stream; there are no surprises there. I can take my shirt off and lie in the sun for hours, cupping my hand into the water and bringing the drops up onto my stomach. I love the heat, the way it burns through my skin. My spot by the stream provides safe seclusion. There's comfort in knowing I'm only a few miles from my house. It's different from being on the remote trail in Alaska. I can be secluded, but I'm only a short ride from a telephone.

I went to the stream to think last summer. To watch the seasons change, watch my own life change. Plagued with the fear of going blind, I wanted to absorb everything with my eyes. Remember the water, the way it looked. I needed to burn the image into my memory to take with me into darkness. But it was really my autonomy I feared losing the most. Not being able to ride my bike there by myself and find my way down the trail to the water. I knew that if my vision went, so would my privacy, my ability to function on my own. I wondered how I would find the will to continue living.

The worries about my health that were whispers when I was growing up now echo loudly in my ears. I can't keep myself from thinking about the future. I try to pretend there's nothing wrong, to go on with my life as it was before the eye problems. I wish I couldn't see the vessels breaking back there, but I'm reminded every time I open my eyes.

I ride hard. My legs burn as the bike picks up speed. The wind always seems to blow twice as hard in the country. My dad always says if it's not at your back, it's against you. An occasional car passes me on this country road, but mostly I'm alone. I ride against the wind. Deserted cornfields push up against the edge of the road, spreading last year's forgotten weeds over the asphalt. The dead fields wait to be given life again.

I thought about suicide a lot last summer. I sat on my lawn chair next to the stream and thought about how I would kill myself if my vision got too bad. I knew the desolate riverbank would be the best place because my parents wouldn't be the ones to find me. I didn't want them living with the image of my dead body in their heads. But then I got worried that maybe no one would find me out there. And I didn't want my father searching ditches across the state as I'd seen parents on television do. I didn't want him to think I'd been kidnapped and lie awake every night worrying about what was happening to me at that moment. My mother has always been paranoid that one of her kids would come up missing.

I was nine years old when a paperboy was kidnapped in Des Moines. Johnny Gosch was delivering the morning newspaper when he disappeared. One of his customers said he'd spotted a white van parked in the shadows. A white van. No real clues. Almost fifteen years later, I still see his pictures on milk cartons and television shows. Artists have aged him in some of the photographs, tried to guess what he might look like now. He's about my age, and his mother is still searching for him.

Brian and I delivered the evening paper the year Johnny Gosch disappeared, and my mother never let us walk the route alone after that. She made us wait until she got home from work. Then she slipped out of her heels and into her tennis shoes and walked with us. Brian argued that he was almost fourteen, but she said she wasn't taking any chances. I heard her talking on the phone with her friends about the missing paperboy. She said she'd rather her children be dead than missing. That way she would just know. I reasoned that I'd have to kill myself someplace where I would be found. I'd want my mom's mind at ease right away. A quick death discovered by strangers. I planned to do it with sleeping pills while the sun beat down on me.

I'd even written the letters to my family and friends. Addressed and stamped. Told them not to be sad, that there was nothing they could have done, that it was my decision. I wanted to die. I wanted to die rather than live blind. I wrote and rewrote the letters. After trying to find the words that fit, I finally settled for excuses I knew would be unacceptable. A letter wouldn't console my mother. Staring at my words, my handwriting, might even make it worse for her. But I couldn't leave the people I loved with no explanation. They deserved to know my reasons.

The letter to my father had been the longest. I wrote that I was sorry, that I knew I was being selfish. I told him I understood that losing two daughters in one lifetime was too much for anyone, but he had to remember me as I had been when I was happier. He loves to see me smile. I wrote that I knew we'd be together again and I would watch over him until then. But eventually that letter fell into selfish excuses too, defending my decision and arguing that it was my choice, my life.

I could never find the right words. I figured they would just come to me when the time was right. I thought I might just wake up one day when my vision was so poor I didn't want to go on, and I would have a moment of clarity. I would know what to write. But my vision hasn't gotten that bad, and I glance up at the clouds as the bike moves me forward. The breeze pushes a strand of hair against my cheek, tickling me. I don't want to die.

We never think we can endure as much as we can. My friend whose kidneys failed told me that. He says he thought about suicide all the time when he was first diagnosed, weighing the quality of his life against the quantity. He never thought he could cope, but he did. After I was diagnosed with retinopathy and feeling hopeless, he told me I was stronger than I gave myself credit for. He said a survival instinct would kick in. When I told him I'd never be able to live blind, he simply responded that I would adjust if it happened. I would redefine what was important in my life. He said I would lose and gain vision, but I still haven't found that optimism.

I pull off the road and follow the railroad tracks about half a mile before arriving at my bridge. Stepping off my bike and walking carefully down the steep hill, I spot my lawn chair wedged between two boards. Warm relief sweeps over me. No one has been here. The chair is exactly where I left it. The nylon seat is torn and the bolts are rusting. The logs I dragged over next to the water are still in place.

I look for a train, craving the familiar rattle on the tracks above. I can always hear them for miles before they arrive, and when they finally make it to the bridge, the ground seems to shake uncontrollably. Sometimes I keep my eyes closed, welcoming the interruption in the silence. If I'm reading, I set my book aside and try to count the cars, but they move too fast. I can hardly differentiate one car from the next. Just a blur of reds and greens. There are no trains here today. Nothing but quiet.

I'm trying to put my life in perspective now. I'm trying to learn to be thankful for my health, rather than resenting a body that has betrayed me. But it's hard to stay focused. Ann graduated from college and works full-time. Holly has a husband and son. I'm busy with graduate school. I find excuses to be by myself. I'm more comfortable when I have no one to compare myself to. If other young bodies aren't parading before me, I can forget that I, too, should be that youthful and healthy.

The water is shallow, beckoning me to plunge my feet down into its muck and let the cold, lumpy mud ooze between my toes. The hot sun beating on my neck almost fools me into believing it's warm enough to remove my socks and shoes. But I resist. Instead I pull my worn sweatshirt over my head and push the hair away from my face. Opening and closing my eyes, I try soaking up the calming silence, but my body refuses to relax. My fingernails dig into the sand beneath me.

Finally I stand up and tie the thin sweatshirt around my waist. I breathe deliberately and deeply. Distinct signs of spring surround me. Birds fly from tree to tree to become familiar with their new homes, and green buds bring life to dark branches. Cool air mixes with warm sun rays. I study my surroundings carefully. My palms start to sweat. I have looked forward to spring for months, but now the chirping birds seem suddenly intrusive. I stand alone on the edge of the stream. Lost. I turn from the water. After pushing my bike up the steep hill, I ride slowly home.

"LONG RIDE?" a voice suddenly comments behind me as I pedal.

The neighbor I was watching earlier pulls up next to me. I look down at his bike and nod. He has interrupted my thoughts. I slow down but don't stop.

"I see you outside all the time," he says, stopping his bike and resting his foot on the curb. I push hard on my brakes out of courtesy. "When I saw you taking off on your bike this morning, I was so jealous I got my own bike out."

Even though the sun glares into his eyes, he looks directly at me as he speaks. His smile is natural, and a bead of sweat rolls down his neck onto the front of his red T-shirt. His thin arms are pale from the long winter, and his cut-off jeans expose the curly hair on his legs. Literally the boy next door. He's hard to resist.

"It's a nice day to ride," I reply. My voice cracks. It's the first time I've spoken today. I look down at his worn tennis shoes.

"I'm Doug," he says, hesitating. "I live across from you." He points down the street to the square, gray house with white shutters.

I follow his gaze and nod. "I saw you this morning. Playing hooky from work?"

He explains that he is a counselor for delinquent teenagers and in between meetings.

"Interesting" escapes my lips. It's the adjective I resort to when I can't find anything else to say.

Our conversation is polite, but I look at my watch repeatedly. He pretends not to notice and continues to talk for several minutes. Then I find myself welcoming the conversation. He tells me stories about his roommate, Craig. He asks me questions about myself and then studies my face, listening intently as I answer.

Cars pass slowly by us. A school bus pulls to a stop at the corner and kids swinging backpacks flood the sidewalk. The sun dips behind a cloud and though the air turns cooler, my body doesn't feel the chill.

Opening My Eyes

I HEAR DOUG opening and shutting the cupboards in the kitchen. He's wondering again why I have so many pots and pans when I rarely cook. During the six years I've lived away from my parents, my mother has given me every kitchen appliance and utensil in the stores. Each Christmas I tear the familiar wrapping paper off the box of an item I've never heard of. My cupboards are filled with iced tea machines, toaster ovens, Ginsu knives, juicers, grinders, choppers, mixers. A special apple peeler. A machine just for potatoes. One spatula for hash browns and another for hamburgers. Pans that steam rice while they cook your vegetables. Then my mom forgets what she's given me and I end up opening an identical box a few years later. I think she worries that it's her fault I didn't turn out to be more domestic.

A pan hits the floor. It's probably Doug's huge aluminum wok. He brought it with him when he moved in and cooks everything in it. He's been living here three weeks now. The neighbors had been eyeing us for months as we walked back and forth across the street to see each other.

Early one morning several weeks after I met him, Doug walked out my back door and straight into our neighbor Dave, who was loading carpet into his van. Doug called me when he got across the street to his house. He was embarrassed but trying to laugh. Dave had looked him up and down twice, from his messed-up hair to his untucked shirt and down to his shoelaces dragging behind his sneakers. He had chuckled and given Doug a knowing look before turning back to his work. When Doug told me it was one of those "man to man" looks, I laughed into the telephone receiver. I knew that we would be the topic of conversation for the next week in the driveways up and down the street.

We walked back and forth across the street for three months before we decided to move in together. Then we tried to devise the most inconspicuous plan for getting his belongings across the street without the neighbors seeing us. At first, we brought one item over at a time. But when we had to move Doug's bed, dresser, and rocking chair, the curtains on our neighbors' windows were pulled back a crack. Even though we had waited until ten o'clock at night to haul the furniture across the street, we could feel their eyes watching us. Doug rolled his eyes when an aluminum pan fell from a box, making a clanging noise that rang through the street. Underwear escaped his laundry basket and landed on the driveway. As we sneaked across the street carrying a mattress, the headlights of Dave's van blinded us. My neighbor pulled into his driveway and asked if we needed some help. Trying to suppress giggles, I replied that Doug and I had it all under control.

At first I didn't want to tell Doug I was diabetic, but he spotted the needles a week after I met him. He was leaning back in the kitchen chair, telling me about his parents. He ran his middle finger around the rim of the coffee mug and stared at the tabletop as he talked. His mom and dad loved to dance, and Doug would stand in the doorway of the kitchen and watch them jitterbug to the music on the radio. Then came the fights. And then the divorce when he was eight. Doug stopped talking and narrowed his eyes when he spotted a needle on the floor next to his chair. The orange cap caught his eye. He looked up at me and back to the needle. *Heroin?* he asked, suddenly smiling. I didn't even have to look down to know what he was referring to. I stared straight into his eyes and confessed that I had been found out.

Like most people, he turned his head when I gave my shots. Sometimes his curiosity got the best of him, and even though he still turned his head, his eyes drifted to the needle in my hand. But the moment the point slipped beneath the surface of my skin, his shoulders tensed up and he looked away.

I told him I was just like everyone else and my eyes were going to get better. I'd had diabetes my entire life and it didn't interfere with anything I did. I convinced him it wasn't a big deal. I'm an expert at that. Few of my friends take the illness seriously, because I never talk about it, never complain about it. Diseases aren't the topic of conversation with my friends. We might share our grandparents' or parents' health problems but rarely our own. When I first developed complications with my eyes, Holly was shocked. She told me she didn't even know that the disease posed a real threat to my health. She thought the only difference between me and her was that I gave shots.

Doug didn't know much about diabetes either, and it wasn't hard to ease his mind. He didn't doubt what I told him about the illness at first, but when he walked through the back door carrying a book on diabetes, I knew I'd have to explain. He pointed to statements on the pages and asked me questions. I took the book from him and pulled the library card from the front pocket. Turning it over in my hand, I looked up at him and answered his questions. Yes, lower-limb amputations are a possibility. Yes, I told him, there is a chance I could go blind. I raised my eyebrows at him as if to say "So what? We all die." I was defensive. Eventually he stopped reading. He said we'd deal with whatever came along. I kept telling him nothing was going to happen to me.

But now he makes lunch while I lie in bed. The doctors in Iowa City performed a vitrectomy on my left eye yesterday. I thought I was prepared this morning as I removed the gauze patch before my bathroom mirror, but I guess nothing could have prepared me for what I saw. Blood covered the entire white of my eye. I look like a demon in a comic book. The surgeon said it would look like someone had punched me, but I think a baseball full of nails thrown at my eye is a more fitting analogy. The lid is so swollen that I had to pry it up with my fingernail to see inside. And when I did get a look, I started crying, yelling for Doug to come and help me put the patch back on. Now I won't take it off. I want to hide from everyone, including myself. I wait in bed for my lunch.

I reach up and place my hand over the patch covering my left eye. The pain is bad, and I feel around on the nightstand for the bottle of pills. They make me sleepy, but sleep is a relief. The emaciated-looking doctor told me not to exceed four tablets a day, but I've already had five since this morning. I know that three times the recommended dosage won't hurt me. Doctors are too careful. Setting the round white pill on the back of my tongue, I take a sip of the water from my glass.

I rest my head back on the pillow and set my hand over my eye again. My fingertips are met with a huge wad of gauze. The doctor used a metal guard around my eye and then wrapped it up with layers of gauze and medical tape to secure it. He told me that it was critical I didn't bump or touch the eye. The eye. Doctors always talk about my eyes like they don't belong to me, like they are in the room with us, but no one wants to claim them. They told me to wear glasses or sunglasses to protect the eye when I'm awake and tape this guard back around the eye every night for the rest of the month. Then put two different drops in the eye four times each day and a creamy salve at night. Dilation drops, an antibiotic, and a steroid. Don't rub the stitches if they start to itch. So many rules.

The surgeon gave me all the details before the surgery.

"I'm recommending a vitrectomy," he began. He was tall with graying hair and bright green eyes. I had seen his picture on the wall in the waiting room, and I knew he was someone important. "You've had more vitreous hemorrhages, and we want to go in and clear the debris out. It's an invasive procedure, so you'll have to stay overnight."

"Are you going to put me under?" I asked.

"Yes. We'll use a general anesthesia." He paused. "I've seen a lot of diabetics in this position. We're thinking about your long-term vision and this is my recommendation. We'll remove the blood-filled vitreous gel and replace it with a saline solution. This won't affect the function of your eye though."

There were about twenty questions running through my head.

"Doesn't my body need that fluid? Is it going to make more?"

"Well"—he hesitated—"it will never make more vitreous gel, but the saline will be absorbed by the system as if it belongs there. The natural gel is much thicker and consequently it's harder for the debris to settle out of your eye. When we remove the vitreous gel, we'll also remove the debris that's in there. You won't see the spiderwebs and shadows you see now."

I knew it couldn't be that simple.

"So it will be completely clear?" I asked.

"Most of it will be cleared out. It's like a glass of dirty water." He picked up a clear plastic cup from the counter next to us. "If there is muddy water in this glass and I dump it out," he said, turning the glass upside down, "there's going to still be some dirt stuck to the sides. Then, when we fill it back up, it will be mostly clear, but probably not completely."

He said they would go in through the sclera, the white of my eye. Small incisions would be made on both sides of my iris and instruments inserted through the front. He must have seen the shock on my face, because he gave me a smile and told me he'd performed hundreds of these operations. He was going to put in a fiberoptic light through one side and a variety of cutters, forceps, and scissors through the other incision. The word *variety* made me nervous. Then he said they would place a microscope over my face to focus through the pupil.

"So what are the risks?" I asked. "Is there a chance I could lose more vision?" I took a deep breath and tried to smile. "I mean what if one of those little pairs of scissors just slips a little bit?"

He pulled up a chair and sat down, moved his head closer to mine.

"In all the years I've performed these, I've had very few problems," he assured me. I knew he was choosing his words carefully. "I have to tell you that vision loss is always a possibility, but, like I said, I've rarely seen it happen. Not from this surgery anyway."

"What about infections?" I asked. I'd heard that once an eye infection starts, it can be hard to control and it usually spreads to the other eye.

"We do everything we can to prevent infections. You'll be using an antibiotic drop in your eye for several weeks following the surgery. And an infection in one eye doesn't affect the other eye."

Then he quickly reminded me that the benefits outweigh the risks. He referred to the vitrectomy as part of the plan. The plan to preserve my vision as best they could. It was never about restoring the vision I'd lost but about preventing losing more.

Two students no older than myself hovered near the door, never looking me in the eye but listening carefully to the surgeon's words. They took notes on what he said to me. They were learning about diabetic eye disease but, more important, learning through the doctor's example how to communicate with patients. I rarely heard a word from any of the students. They were trained to be quiet and ask their questions outside the examination rooms. I knew they had to learn somewhere.

I stared at the students hard, wanting them to look up at me, remember what I was like when I was awake. I wanted them to see my eyes when they were part of a whole person, not just a face under a microscope. I thought having them all in surgery would make me more comfortable, but I was struck with a fear of an argument breaking out between them in the operating room if they didn't agree on something. Debating about what to do next as I lay unconscious. I knew that this man in a white coat doing all the talking was in charge. Later that day I found out he was the head of retina surgery. He would perform the surgery, another doctor would assist him, and the students would watch. I had gotten used to several pairs of eyes staring through lenses at my blood vessels by then.

"What's the alternative?" I asked.

He pressed his lips together. "We can wait and see how the eye behaves. We would definitely have to go in and add more laser to the eye very soon, something we would be able to go ahead and do while you were having the vitrectomy if you decide to take that route. The alternative is to wait and see if that debris will clear out on its own."

"What about afterwards?" I asked. "Is it going to be painful?"

The doctor told me there would be some pain and the eye would be swollen. Then he studied my eyes. Not through a microscope or light but with his naked eyes. It was like he was looking at the color of them rather than the vessels behind the eye. He was looking at me instead of just my weakened nerves. His eyes were telling me that I could trust him. I could let him carry the burden of worrying about the condition during the surgery. Then he pressed his lips together and flipped a light on, pulling the photographs of my retina out of a manila folder.

"See how the red is clouding this area here," he said, pointing to the areas of hemorrhage with his pen. "There have been several breaks back there, and it's going to take quite a while for that to settle out of there. We'll remove this." He circled the pen around the bloody area. "The bottom line is you should see better, Andrea."

That's all I wanted. To see things more clearly, and if a vitrectomy would do that, that's what I wanted too. While I was under, they planned to do a few other things to my left eye.

Adding more laser would save me the discomfort of having to undergo another one of those procedures separately. This would make my seventh laser surgery, the fourth on my left eye. I wondered how many more there would be, but I knew the doctor couldn't answer that question. He said another laser was necessary for now. He wanted to reduce the traction and pulling from new blood vessels and scar tissue. The previous laser surgeries had caused the peripheral vessels in my eye to shrivel up. This is what they wanted to accomplish, but when these vessels became smaller, tension was put on the other vessels near the middle of my retina. The center of the eye was beginning to bulge out and leak fluid into my central vision, causing me to look at the world through a cloud. The doctor wanted the lasered vessels to shrink, but when they do traction occurs. It's a no-win situation, but they always offer the hope that something might improve, the swelling might diminish.

It all sounded too good to be true. Suck the dirty vitreous fluid out and put clean solution back in. I figured the pain would be worth it. I thought I was prepared.

Today I'm not so sure. I keep my right eye shut, waiting for the pain medication to kick in. The floor creaks near the doorway of the bedroom. Doug stands before me with a new gauze patch and tape. I slowly shake my head.

"Come on, Andie. I'll just put the drops in and put the new patch on."

I tilt my head back, surrendering.

Doug carefully pulls the patch off my face. He exhales loudly when he sees the blood, but he doesn't say anything. My right eye follows his hand as he holds a tube of gooey salve over my face. I want to reach up and wipe the muck out of my eye, but I'm afraid to touch it. He takes a sterile gauze pad from a package and places it over my eye, sets the guard on top of that, and tapes it gently to my head. He looks closely at his work. Tears are falling from my right eye and he wipes them away with his thumb. He looks sad.

"Sweetie," he says, gently pressing the tape down. He runs his fingers slowly through my hair, pushing it away from my face.

"It just looks so gross. I look gross," I say, my chest getting tighter.

"It's been less than twenty-four hours. It's going to look better and better each day."

I try to believe him, but there is fear in his voice. We both know it might take weeks for the swelling to go down and possibly months until the blood is cleared. The waiting is the worst part. I wonder how long it will be until I look normal again, until I can see clearly. The doctors can never give me definite answers, only statistics and the stories of cases they're familiar with. Every time I leave the office, a doctor says *we'll* wait a month and I should come back then. But I'm the one who waits; it's not something they do with me. When I walk out of there, they move to their next patient, and I am the one who waits every night for something to get better or worse. I am the one who gets up each morning and waits for a vessel to break, forcing me to rearrange my day. This morning the doctors told me that we'd have to wait and see how long recovery time will be.

"I'll get your lunch," Doug says, pushing himself off the bed.

I can feel his anxiety. He's afraid of losing me, nervous about my diabetes. I think the shock of seeing me lying in the hospital bed last night scared him. Like people in hospital beds inevitably die. He sat next to my bed all night, resting his head on my stomach. I keep waiting for his fear to drive him away from me, but it doesn't.

"You okay in there?" Doug yells down the hall.

"Yup," I yell back, my head pounding furiously.

He walks back into the bedroom carrying a big plate in one hand and a glass in the other. He places the dishes on the nightstand and pulls a napkin, a needle, insulin, and a fork from his shirt pocket. He's made spaghetti.

"You're such a good nurse," I reassure him.

He smiles and slides into bed next to me, grabs the remote

control, and turns the television volume down. He bends the pillow in half and shoves it against the headboard. Then he pauses before he leans back. He reaches up and grabs the napkin off the nightstand, tucking a corner into the collar of my T-shirt. My eye follows him as he leans close to me and settles into the pillow. His lips are perfectly curved, and his bottom teeth are crooked. I wonder which one of his parents he looks like.

I think I'm finally accepting his help, his presence. I'd been alone for so long before I met him, going through the motions of each day and rarely thinking about the romantic future. Even when I first started spending a lot of time with him, I never imagined we'd be living together. I thought I was destined to be alone like my sister. It wasn't as though I thought having diabetes made me a liability to someone else, but I just didn't think I'd live very long. I didn't think I was going to be around to have kids and retire.

"Why don't you go out with Craig tonight?" I ask. "I'll be okay here and you need to get out."

He looks hurt. "You want to be alone?"

"No," I say. "I'm just afraid you're going to get tired babysitting me and my patch." I try to smile.

He puts his arms around me, but I pull away. He tries to hold me tighter as I stare through my right eye at the ceiling. The napkin falls to the floor. I reach up and touch my patch again.

"Are you going to eat?" he asks.

"Yeah," I reply, making no move to pick up the plate.

I turn to face him, letting him examine the patch on my eye without moving my head away. I force my right eye open wide. My left eye stirs beneath the patch. He runs his finger down my right cheek, carefully studying my expression. I want to cry again, but I can't let myself. All the tears only make my eyes smaller and more swollen. If I cry any more, I won't be able to see at all.

I don't really expect Doug to understand how I'm feeling. I

tried to explain to him what the world looked like to me since my eyes have gotten bad. A few weeks ago, I punched about twenty holes in a sheet of notebook paper and held it in front of his face. I told him to look through it. Spots. I told him I saw black spots where objects used to be. He frowned and nodded before taking the paper from my hand. He laid it carefully on the coffee table and wrapped his arms around me. I don't expect him to understand any more than that. I can describe the condition, but I can never explain how I feel about it. I'm alone in this. No one can understand how fearful I am of going blind, how secluded I am in my thoughts about my future.

"I'm tired," I say, letting my head fall back on the pillow.

He says nothing but positions himself more tightly around me. I let him. His hand rests on my stomach and I trace the outline of his fingers with mine. Soft hands. They are young compared to mine. I'm self-conscious about the wrinkles on my fingers, and I tighten my hand into a fist and slip it under his. I've had the hands of an old woman since I was a child. My mother used to tell me they were wise, told me I inherited them from my grandmother. Just forty years too soon, I replied. I loosen my fist and feel his fingers closing around mine. He holds on for his life. For my life. Like if he lets me go even for a moment, I might slip away.

Healing Touch

F ifteen years," I tell the old woman. "I was diagnosed when I was nine." She's sitting too close to me on the over-stuffed couch.

"And you're on insulin?" she asks, studying my face. Her voice is almost a whisper. Her eyes are dark and her body is plump from age.

I nod and look around the room. She's transformed the attic of her Dutch Colonial house into an office. The room is dark except for the glow from the votive candles bouncing off the slanted walls. The bookshelves are lined with porcelain animals and books on alternative medicine. I have some of the same books at home on the art of relaxation, how to heal the body naturally, and acupuncture. My books talk about healers like this woman. Black leaves smolder in a small hand-painted bowl on the table in front of us. A smell of spices and pine permeates the room.

"You know this isn't a replacement for your traditional doctors," she says, finally inching a comfortable distance away from me. "Healing touch is a complement to your insulin and diet. The something extra that gives you the edge over other diabetics. The mind can heal the body. The mind is stronger than the body."

I know her therapy can't replace my insulin injections, but I want to believe that she can do something for me the doctors can't. Maybe teach me how to do more for myself. Holly calls her the healing woman, says she's heard the old lady has a special gift. My friend told me yesterday that I should let the woman work on me, but I need to believe in order for the sessions to help me. I stare down at my sister's class ring on my pinkie.

"I've been through several laser surgeries on my eyes, and sometimes my feet go numb. I can feel tingling in my legs when I wake up in the morning." I'm telling her things I wouldn't even say to Dr. Manning.

She nods and asks if I take any vitamins.

"Yes," I reply. I know about vitamins.

"What are you taking?" She looks genuinely interested.

"E, C, B-complex, lecithin, flaxseed oil, calcium, and selenium."

She is impressed, so I continue.

"The E is for circulation. I take the C for my immune system, the B-complex because I'm a vegetarian. Lecithin aids in breaking down cholesterol, and I just started taking flaxseed oil because I read that it can help people with diabetic retinopathy. Calcium I need because I don't drink milk or eat many dairy products, and the selenium is to aid in the utilization of vitamin E." I exhale and settle back into the thick cushion.

My dad's been taking vitamins for years. He's told me stories about the acne he was afflicted with throughout adolescence and into his twenties. He visited all the doctors in Des Moines and washed his face three or four times a day. Nothing worked. Finally a friend gave him an article about vitamin A, and he started consuming megadoses. He said he took what are now considered to be toxic doses of the vitamin, but the acne cleared. Years of scarring disappeared in less than a month. He never had another skin problem, and he became a strong advocate of vitamins, suggesting this or that one whenever a family friend complained about a health problem. He thinks vitamins can help everyone.

I took my first vitamins when I was eleven. It was a Saturday morning, and I woke up before my parents. Brian was with a friend, so the house was quiet. I flipped on the small television on the kitchen counter and sat down to a breakfast of saltines. My dad had left an article on the kitchen table about diabetics benefiting from vitamin E. It had saved them from amputations, healed sores on their feet, and cured blindness. My dad collected all the articles on vitamins and diabetes for my sister. He tucked them in folders according to the vitamin. They were alphabetized from "Vitamin A" to "Zinc" in the file cabinet downstairs. Munching on my crackers, I read the article on the table carefully. The childlike voices of cartoon characters wailed on the screen. The article said vitamin E was a great preventative vitamin, so I dug through the kitchen cupboard and found a big brown bottle. Pouring twenty or thirty capsules into my hands, that morning's breakfast became orange juice, crackers, and the capsules of vegetable oil. Within ten minutes, my stomach was heaving.

My dad walked into the bathroom, saw me leaning over the toilet, and put his hand on my back. His light blue pajama bottoms brushed the tops of his feet. He asked me if I had the flu. When I confessed what I'd done, he rubbed his tired eyes and smiled. He said it sounded like I'd gone a little overboard. I looked back down into the toilet and agreed. That afternoon he bought me my own bottles at the drugstore and cleared a shelf in the kitchen cabinet for me, just my vitamins. He gave me a small notebook of articles from *Prevention* magazine and a book written by Adele Davis. Taking the pills became a ritual, something my dad and I did together. We set our orange, white, and yellow tablets next to our plates at the table. When he swallowed his, I swallowed mine.

My sister took vitamins her entire life. The brown bottles filled a shelf in our bathroom closet. She always said diabetics were deficient and complications were probably related to the deficiencies. She took handfuls of the pills, claiming she would get sick if she skipped a day. The last few years she was alive, she took more, since cocaine depletes the system of nutrients. Denise would even puncture the end of a vitamin E capsule with a needle and squeeze the gel on her finger, push the goop up into her nose. Cocaine irritates the nasal passages, and she said vitamin E soothes them.

I don't tell the healing woman the stories of my family, even though I know she would listen. She's leaning closer to me again, staring into my eyes.

"You can't see them," I inform her. I know what she's looking for. "Only I can see the breaks. They're behind the lens." I'm used to people gazing into my eyes when I tell them I have retinopathy. They crane their necks forward and move their heads back and forth slowly, searching for anything out of the ordinary.

She nods but continues to look.

Then she explains to me that what she does is similar to religion. She relies heavily on faith, on healing the body through using the mind. The woman covers her eyes with her hands and tells me to do the same. I stare at the deep wrinkles lining her knuckles. No rings. Then I cover my own eyes. She tells me to imagine I'm healing the weak blood vessels. Get a visual of them and repair them in my mind. She tells me to conjure an image in my head of one of the microscopic blood vessels, make it very large, and work around it slowly, repairing it as I go. I should be able to see it all.

I'm afraid to peek out from under my hands. I can feel her watching me. I sit for several minutes, trying to concentrate, waiting to hear the sound of her voice again. The smell of the leaves is more prominent now. I can't visualize a blood vessel. I only know what the pictures of my retina look like and how the black lines and spots look after the vessel has hemorrhaged. An image of a small capillary flashes in my mind for a moment. I try to recapture it, but I can't. I stay still and quiet. Finally the woman speaks, telling me I can open my eyes now. She says I should do this every day. Imagine I am healing myself, trust that I have the power to cure my condition.

Then she pulls a book from a basket on the floor and opens it up to a drawing of a woman standing over a half-clothed child. The healer. The figures are sketched in gray, but blue and yellow streams of light connect the healer's hands to the patient's body. The small child's eyes are closed, and the healer is looking toward the sky. There's a chill in this room, and I want to ask if I'm going to have to take off my clothes too. The woman seems to read my mind—she informs me that she won't touch me. She says her fingers will never make contact with my skin as she gets my energy fields back in balance. She explains when there's something wrong on the inside, the energy on the outside has holes in it. She will bring the broken energy back together, make it whole again.

"Go ahead and make yourself comfortable up there," she says, motioning to the table in the middle of the room. It looks like a hospital gurney with a white sheet draping over the sides. I lean forward and slip my shoes off before pushing myself off the couch. The woman doesn't move. I climb onto the table and lie flat on my back like the child in the picture. I close my eyes and listen for the woman. Her knees crack and I can feel her moving toward me. Hovering above me. I try to imagine blue energy broken up above my body, but I can't stay focused. I want to open my eyes, see what she's doing. If she's looking to the sky like the woman in the picture, she won't catch me looking at her.

I contemplate whether I should open my eyes or not for several minutes. I know I'm not focused as I should be. I'm supposed to be thinking about my body and about the healing process. Finally I open my left eye a crack. Through my eyelashes, I see her moving slowly around my torso. Her head is tilted to the ceiling, moving to a rhythm I don't hear. Her eyes are closed. Just like the picture. She's moving her hands in circles about two inches above my stomach. I close my eyes again.

There's a part of me that wants to dismiss alternative therapies as a hoax. When I told Doug I was coming here today, he narrowed his eyes and asked why. I knew he was classifying this woman with tarot card readers and Dionne Warwick. I simply told him that I had to try this woman, partly out of desperation and partly out of curiosity. I needed to talk about my health to someone who didn't wear a white coat and hold a clipboard. Doug shrugged his shoulders.

Doug believes only in what he can see. He says that his experiences are real and he can't believe in things he can't touch. He understands the concept of faith but can't accept it for himself. I tell him there's more to the world than what's right here in front of us. I have to believe that. It keeps me sane. He replies that it's just hard for human beings to imagine the world without them in it. We're anthropocentric and scared to think of our own nonexistence, so we create beliefs out of fear.

My parents weren't religious. My father was raised a staunch Catholic but fell from faith in his late twenties. He was excommunicated when he married my mother and she refused to convert. She said she wouldn't promise anyone that she would raise her kids to believe something she didn't believe in. My parents told me faith is internal. Believe in things, but don't be limited by them. Explore everything because you stop living when you adhere too strongly to any one thing. Don't be controlled by what you're told to do, but, rather, control what you do by going on your instinct for what's right.

They taught me to always be open to new possibilities, and I guess that's why I'm here on this table. The practice of healing is as old as religion. Even the Bible records faith healing. I'm not a Christian, but the stories of Jesus healing the blind intrigue me. Later, healing powers were assigned to kings who claimed to be able to heal through "royal touch." Some people even claim that healing energy can stimulate plants to grow and quicken the healing of wounds on rats. The stories of the Bible were stories, and kings were only men born to the right mother. But there's something I believe about all this, something I need to believe.

I bought a book on yoga several weeks ago. I lit a candle and sat in the middle of my living room floor, glancing at the book every time I wanted to switch poses. It looked so easy in the pictures. The stretching and breathing calmed me, but then when I moved into the more complex positions I got distracted. I tried to balance my weight on my hands and twist my legs behind my back. Doug was at work, and I knew he would be laughing if he was home. I resorted to the headstand. I knew I could do that one. I closed my eyes, leaned forward, and pushed my legs into the air. The blood rushed to my head. I counted twenty-five deep breaths while I focused on keeping my balance. Then when I sat up, I saw the blood in my right eye. All the debris was floating around behind the lens. I slid the book underneath the coffee table and turned on the television.

A friend at school suggested acupuncture, an ancient medical system that originated in China and espouses preventative medicine, keeping the body well. In China, patients used to pay the doctor as long as they were in good health and stopped paying him when they became ill. Acupuncturists believe we each possess a finite amount of energy called *chi*. This energy is our life force, and we can increase its circulation by taking good care of ourselves or deplete the energy through stress and poor nutrition. Illness is a deficiency or excess of our *chi*, and the needles used in acupuncture can slow down, speed up, or unblock stuck energy. I've thought about visiting an acupuncturist, but I'm not sure about letting someone besides me stick needles into my skin.

I'll see how I feel after today. This woman seems honest. She looks peaceful too, possessing a certain inner strength. At least sixty years old, she doesn't have the harried look that many older people do. She has lived alone in the same house for the last thirty-five years, and she still delivers mail for the post office every day. She told me she loves her job because she gets to put the news of the world into mailboxes. Bringing them joy and pain in white envelopes.

My legs are getting warmer, and I know without looking that her hands are hovering above my knees. I am surprised by the hot sensation, but I keep my eyes closed, trying to concentrate on the energy. My mind wanders. She told me that people describe their experiences with her differently. Some claim that their entire body tingles, others say they feel like they are in a deep trance, and some admit that they feel nothing. Don't go to sleep, she said to me. She told me she'd know if I did and would gently shake me to keep me semialert. It's important that I remain conscious in order to participate in this session. She said that both of us have to concentrate for it to work. I focus on my thighs.

After what seems like minutes, I feel her fingers on my shoulder. The contact feels impersonal now.

"Do you know how long you've been lying here?" she asks.

I think for a moment, trying to calculate passed time. There are no clocks on the walls in here.

"Twenty-five minutes?" I ask.

"Almost two hours," she replies.

"Is there that much work to be done on me?" I laugh.

She smiles. "Well, you have a lot of fragmented energy. I tried to do some overall repair this first time, getting your energy field back in flow."

She gently eases me up into a sitting position on the table.

"Your energy is fragmented in your lower limbs and fingertips," she tells me. Her head is tilted to the side and she looks like she just woke up.

I wonder if she would have come up with this same diagnosis if I hadn't told her that my feet sometimes go numb. On my drive over here, I contemplated not revealing any information about my health to her. I thought this would be a fair test to see if she was for real. But I was overcome with a sense of trust when I saw her, and I didn't want to deceive her. I wanted her to work with me.

"And my eyes?" I ask. "Did you detect anything wrong in my eyes?"

"No, but I tried to stay away from that area. I don't want to add lasers of my own quite yet. If you decide you want to come back for another session, we'll talk about targeting your eyes for special work. Energy lasers are very powerful, and I'll need to caution you about that process before we start."

I FEEL exhaustion mixed with a sense of peace as I walk across the lawn to my car. I'm not sure what I'll tell Doug. I turn the key in the ignition and sit back in my seat. The seat belt light on the dash flashes. I take deep breaths and try to hold on to the calm. More than anything, I feel rested. The lights in the healing woman's living room go off. I didn't see a television or radio or computer anywhere in her house, but I didn't detect loneliness in her eyes either. I wonder how long she can stand being alone in this brick house on the east side of Des Moines. All the windows in the elementary school across the street are dark. Perhaps the neighborhood children fear her, call her a witch, and dare each other to walk across her porch after dark.

My skin tingles as I put my car in drive and creep slowly past her house. Glancing at the clock on my radio, I realize that it has been almost three hours since I left my house. Doug is probably waiting for me, wondering how long it takes to be healed. I wonder the same thing. I should feel in control. The healing woman told me over and over that I had the power within me, but I don't have the discipline to concentrate the way she does. Maybe I've relied on the doctors too much, expected them to just fix me. The woman talked about healing, but I want to be fixed. I want to just be fine.

I drive the fifteen minutes back to my house in silence. No familiar sound of the radio blaring in my ears. The healing woman said we have too many distractions. Our society separates us from ourselves, makes it hard to focus on what's important. She told me I should make time for quiet every day. I pull into my driveway and stare at the back of Doug's car. The kitchen light is on.

I push the car door closed softly and tiptoe onto the back deck. Doug is making dinner inside. I stand still and watch him for several minutes as he moves about the kitchen, setting two plates and a bowl of salad on the table. Sidney is staring at him too, waiting for him to drop a scrap of food on the floor. Doug puts ice in two glasses and stares at them for a moment, probably wondering if the frozen water will melt before I come through the door. Looking at his watch, he takes a step toward the window to wash his hands in the sink. I stand in the darkness and feel the cool spring breeze on the back of my neck. I want him to see me now, but I don't tap on the glass. Instead, I reach for the doorknob. I am home.

To Be a Woman

THE ANESTHESIOLOGIST wraps a blood pressure cup around my arm. I stare at the IV needle deep in my hand and wonder if I'm the youngest person they've performed this procedure on here. Maybe they coddle everyone the way they did me this morning, wrapping me in a blanket and placing me in a plush recliner. But I think they treated me so well because I'm younger than most of the women who come through their doors. Women several years older than myself who are confident in their decisions not to have any more children. Maybe they were so gentle because they felt sorry for me. One of the nurses sat down next to me and asked me how many children I have. When I replied that I didn't have any, she nodded her head and pulled the blanket up around my chin. I wanted to explain to her that this is my decision, my choice.

Doug is in the waiting room listening to whatever morning talk show is playing on the television. He is probably thumbing through the files in his briefcase, reviewing the cases of distraught teenagers. Kids who use drugs and run away from home. I find myself hoping that all the kids he works with will somehow kill his desire to have a family of his own. I think that maybe he'll get discouraged seeing all their problems and decide that it's better we don't have any ourselves. But he doesn't. His work only makes him more confident that he can be the right kind of parent. He says he knows which mistakes to try to avoid making. He wants children, but he's still here with me today.

The man above me attaches heart monitors to my chest and talks to the nurse next to him about his plans for the upcoming Fourth of July weekend. He and his wife will be taking their children to watch fireworks.

"You know how Chelsea is," he says. "The little monster will run straight at a bottle rocket to try to catch the damn thing."

"She is a character," the nurse replies.

They've forgotten I'm here.

"So no more of that this year," he says. He's decided not to drive down to Missouri and buy fireworks for his family this summer. It's safer to watch them from across a field somewhere. Keep their distance.

I'll never have children. I'm more afraid now than I was as a teenager. I've heard the stories of pregnant diabetic women who have gone blind or lost their kidneys. Even when I hear about successful diabetic pregnancies, I dismiss those women as lucky. Exceptions to the rule. The risks to my health aren't worth it. So I'm here to undergo the surgery to make sure I never get pregnant. The surgery that ultimately makes my decision for me in case I ever get any crazy ideas about changing my mind. Lying on my back in this white room, I wonder if I'm doing this because I don't trust myself, or doing it to prove to Doug that there is really no hope of its ever happening. I want to be sure he knows that I'm never going to change my mind. That after today we *can't* change our minds. He needs to know the truth, because he asked me to marry him one month ago on a hot June afternoon.

We had been bike riding all day and stopped at my stream to rest. The mosquitoes were biting my arms and I kept telling him I wanted to go back home, but he insisted that we stay just a few minutes longer. Even though we were sitting in the shade, sweat was dripping down my sunburned cheeks, and I wiped perspiration from the backs of my knees. I kept looking at him, wondering why we couldn't just ride back home and relax in the air-conditioning for the rest of the afternoon. The serious expression on his face made me nervous.

Then I saw the box. He pulled a black leather ring box from his backpack and fell on one knee without looking at me. When he took the ring out, it slipped from his fingers, falling into the sand. His hands were shaking as he picked it up and wiped it on his sweaty T-shirt. Then he held the ring out and told me I was the person he wanted to spend his life with. The air was still and a train chugged in the distance. The diamond sparkled in the sun. I just stared at him as the words tumbled from his lips. He promised to make me happy, said he wanted to grow old with me. Without a word, I held out my hand and he slipped the ring over my sweaty finger.

Tears collected beneath my sunglasses as we rode home that day. I let myself fall behind so he wouldn't see me crying. They weren't tears of happiness, even though I wanted to marry him more than I'd ever wanted to do anything. The tears came from somewhere deep inside me. I was crying because I wanted to grow old with him too, but I knew I wouldn't. I cried because I envied the elderly couples I saw holding hands in the park. I was jealous of their years together, years I believed Doug and I would never have.

I've tried to explain this feeling that I'm going to die young to a few of my friends. They don't really understand; they tell me I shouldn't worry. Ann says that thinking like that will drive me crazy, and any one of us could die at any time. There are no guarantees. She says I can live as long as anyone if I take care of myself. I've heard that all my life from doctors, but I never believe the words. I can't envision myself living past forty. When Denise died, I just accepted that I would probably die in my early thirties as well. Now I just keep quiet about the lingering thoughts of my own mortality. People don't like to hear that kind of talk, but I know the statistics. My body will never last as long as the bodies of my friends. And I won't have kids. Doug needs to accept that.

Coming here to undergo a tubal ligation is the only way I know how to be totally honest with Doug, to make real for him that the decision is final. Dr. Valone stressed the permanence of the procedure, reminding me several times that it was irreversible. He questioned me for a long time as I sat in his office. He even made me think about it for a week and come back and talk to him again before he would schedule a surgery. He showed me a video and told me that diabetes wasn't an excuse not to have my own kids. He said that Type I's can have healthy babies. It's not like it was ten years ago. They monitor diabetic mothers very closely now, regulating their blood sugars hourly. But he couldn't convince me. I'm scared about my health. Scared I won't live to see a child grow up. Nothing he said could make me change my mind. I know that pregnancy can cause complications with my eyes. There are risks. So a tubal ligation is my insurance policy against myself. Sterilization is virtually 100 percent effective.

Dr. Valone said that he hoped I had thought about what a tubal ligation meant for the future. The doctor reminded me that I might decide I want children when I'm thirty-five. Your life is going to change, he told me. Your priorities will be different in ten years. He asked me what Doug wanted. I lied and said that we had worked it all out between us. The doctor believed me when I told him that neither of us wanted kids. But it isn't that simple.

I THOUGHT for a long time about how I would tell Doug I wanted to have my tubes tied. I stood in front of the bathroom mirror and rehearsed the words, trying to anticipate his response. I thought maybe I could scare him with horror stories of pregnant diabetics. Scare him into being the one to suggest I have the surgery done. I stood in front of the mirror and talked, convincing myself with my own words. Then just when I thought I had the right approach, I'd step into the living room and say nothing.

I waited. Weeks passed. Finally, one afternoon as I heard Doug talking on the phone to his sister, I knew it was time. When I heard him say "not right away," I knew she had asked about kids. After he hung up the phone, I just stared at him.

"Not right away?" I asked. "Kids?"

"Yeah," he replied. "It's just that question everyone asks." His tone was passive. Thinking the conversation was finished, he turned around and headed for the kitchen.

"Well, you better tell them," I said. He stopped but didn't turn around. "Let your brother pass down the name."

"I guess they'll just figure it out. Eventually." He still wouldn't face me.

I studied him as he hesitated with his back to me. His wallet was starting to wear through the back pocket of his pants. His shoes were spotless and his waist was thin. The sun coming through the window made his hair look almost blond.

"I'm going to get a tubal ligation," I said.

I couldn't have said those words if he'd been looking at me. The innocence of his light brown eyes always makes me think twice about what I say to him. I couldn't have stated my intentions so matter-of-factly if he'd been facing me. His body stiffened when my words registered.

"What?" he asked, finally turning around.

"I talked to the doctor about it. I don't even have to stay in the hospital overnight. It's a pretty simple procedure."

He continued to stare at me in disbelief.

"Really. I can be in and out of there in a few hours. After that I'll just be sore for a few days, but they do so many of them now, there aren't many risks." I knew I was taking the attention off the issue by focusing on the procedure.

"You talked to a doctor about it?" He raised his eyebrows

and leaned forward. "You talked to a doctor before we talked about it?"

"We *have* talked about it," I said.

Doug didn't know how to respond. I knew he was searching for some memory of this conversation. Finally, he found his voice.

"You mentioned it. Once, I think," he replied. "But I wouldn't call it a mutual decision we've made. I can't believe you talked to the doctor."

"Did you think I was just going to cross my fingers and hope I never get pregnant? I told you I wasn't having kids, and I thought you understood."

He held up his hand.

"Let me get this straight," he said. "You went and consulted with some doctor about whether or not we, you and me"—he pointed his finger at my chest and then his own—"were ever going to have children. You talked to him about one of the biggest decisions in our life without even telling me you were going?"

"I—" I began, but he didn't let me finish.

"Then you made this decision all on your own and you're just letting me in on it now?" He slowly let all the air out of his lungs. "I can't believe this."

I looked down at my shoelaces. I should have prepared myself for a response like that.

"Did you even plan on asking me?" he asked. His voice had risen. "In all your deep contemplation about this decision, did you once stop and consider asking me what I wanted to do?"

And then it turned into an argument. An argument where he called me selfish and I called him selfish and we didn't talk about the issue again the rest of the week. He knew I had scheduled the procedure and he took the day off work. On the way here this morning, I told him I was nervous.

"Don't worry," he said, reaching over and taking my hand. "It'll work out fine."

I wanted to ask him if he was talking about the tubal ligation or our relationship.

"I'm nervous too," he continued.

"About what?" I asked, knowing this was going to be the conversation we should have had weeks ago.

"That you're not thinking this through, and we're going to regret it."

"I did think it through. I've been thinking it through for years. For years before I met you," I replied.

He was silent for several minutes after that. He focused on the traffic, stared intently at stop signs and buildings.

"I just wonder if you still would have done it if I'd asked you not to," he finally said. "If I told you it was important to me and I had asked you to wait, would you have waited?"

I felt I was being asked a loaded question. And the answer I gave would be even more loaded. If I said yes, I was putting his dreams before my health. If I said no, I would be selfish. He was asking me to choose between my loyalty to him and my loyalty to myself. I didn't think I could have it both ways. And if I said nothing, it would be worse. I chose my words carefully.

"If I thought it meant that much to you, I would have waited. I just didn't see the sense in waiting."

He nodded but didn't reply.

"Here?" he asked, pointing to a three-story white building.

"Yes." The clinic loomed before us.

"It just seems like this whole thing is out of my hands," he said as he turned the steering wheel. "Like you just expect me to sit back and accept whatever you do and not say a word."

I wanted to defend myself, but I let him talk.

"I've been thinking about this every day," he continued. "And I think maybe this is an easier decision for you to make." He paused, knowing he needed to soften the blow of his words. "I mean you've had a lifetime to get used to the idea of not having kids. I've had three weeks." He took a deep breath.

I listened carefully to his words, listened to the person

behind his words. I wanted to reach out to him, but I couldn't move. I stared out the window.

"I'm not trying to make this harder on you. I just want you to understand," he said.

I could feel him staring at the back of my head. He touched my hair. I thought about the kind of father he would be, how much pride he would take in his children. I was taking away his opportunity to love our child. I turned my head to him and saw that his expression had softened. He looked defeated.

"Come on, sweetie. Let's go in," he said.

I wanted to sit there for a few more minutes. I wiped my eyes with the back of my sleeve.

"I need to do this, Doug," I said.

He didn't respond, so I picked up the pamphlet I had received from the doctor and concentrated on that. I pretended to read it, even though I had studied it carefully several times already. It explained the tubal ligation procedure, and I held on to it tightly as Doug jingled his keys in his hand. Finally, I wrapped my fingers around the handle on the door and pulled.

I wasn't afraid of the surgery as I walked from the car to the door of the clinic. I wasn't thinking about complications or the scalpel. I wasn't even contemplating my future with Doug. Instead I thought about my mother as I glanced at my reflection in the windows of the clinic. I realized that I would never experience what she had experienced when she gave birth to me and my brother and sister. I thought about never feeling the unconditional love that mothers have for their children. Then I thought about my sister and what her death had done to my parents. They've never been the same. I opened the door to the office and stepped inside.

The doctor is going to fill my abdomen with carbon dioxide gas so he can see the tubes more clearly. The nurse told me that my shoulders might hurt for a few days afterward, but not to worry. The gas is just going to move around my body in an attempt to escape. It's normal, she said. So I close my eyes and try to envision my abdomen blown up. The more I relax, the larger it gets, finally seeming to become larger than my body. I am hovering above myself in a trance. Then I imagine two hands trying to cut through the skin on my stomach, but the flesh has become tough like an orange peel. In this vision, my skin is transparent and I can see the tubes floating around inside. Waiting. But the doctor can't get through to them. I open my eyes.

The ceiling is white and I try to focus on the anesthesiologist. He has finally stopped talking to the nurse and catches me looking at him.

"Feeling okay?" he asks.

My head moves up and down even though I'm not feeling much of anything. It's like the shell of my body is floating in empty space. I long for sleep, but fight against it.

"You'll be awake again before you know it," he reassures me.

I hope he's right, and I hope I don't regret my decision.

I read that over a third of the women who choose sterilization regret it. For some women it's a good thing, but those who do it before the age of thirty are often sorry. The book I read included the testimonies of women who felt they were pressured to undergo a tubal by their husbands or physicians. Some of the women wrote that they didn't feel like women anymore, and they were scared their husbands wouldn't love them. I read about women throughout history who had been deceived by doctors who cut their tubes without their consent. Black women in the South knew a tubal ligation as a "Mississippi appendectomy." After they gave birth to a baby, a doctor would cut and tie their tubes without the woman's knowledge. Some of these women would wonder for years why they could never get pregnant again, finally being told by another physician that they had been sterilized. The book said that women all over the world had been victims of sterilization abuse. If a doctor decided a woman was mentally unfit, he could perform the procedure against her will. There are documented cases of tubal ligations being performed during abortions. Sometimes the doctors wouldn't perform the abortion unless the woman agreed to sterilization as well. Other times, they didn't tell the women what they had done.

I feel a connection to the women I've read about. Even though the decision I'm making is my own, I understand their emotions. I understand their concerns about their husbands' reactions or not feeling completely like a woman afterward. I can even imagine the anger of being coerced and deceived. It's just that I feel deceived by my own body. I thought about these women all week while I waited for this appointment, hoping that I wouldn't feel regret the next year or ten years later. And I hope now that I won't want something I can't have after today.

I would love to leave the world knowing there was still going to be a piece of me behind. Maybe a little girl for Doug to hold on to when I'm gone. She would have brown hair and green eyes, and he could tell her stories about me. She would keep me alive for him and give him someone else to live for. Having a child would give me the peace I might need someday when I die. I could go knowing my husband wouldn't be alone. But I guess I am selfish. I want the world to belong to me.

The doctor interrupts my thoughts. He rests his hand on the side of the thin mattress.

"Hi, Andrea," he says. "Getting sleepy?"

I force a smile. It's almost time, and I know in a few more minutes I'll be asleep. He doesn't need to ask me if I'm sure about my decision now. I've signed the consent forms and I'm ready to do it.

But a conversation I had with Doug a few weeks ago flashes into my mind. He remarked that maybe the scientists would find a cure for diabetes someday. If that happened, I might not be afraid to have children. I replied that there would never be a cure. I wouldn't bet my life on hope. They've been saying there was a cure in sight ever since I could remember, ever since my father could remember. A breakthrough in diabetes means a new way to give an injection or monitor blood sugars. I'm not holding my breath.

A cure for diabetes. I don't even think about that. I just hope for advances in how to treat the complications of the disease. Ways to prevent blindness and restore circulation. A kidney transplant without a life of immunosuppressants. I don't think this is hoping for too much, but a cure is too much to ask for. The doctors say diabetes is manageable, so the focus is on the best ways to manage it. Controlling it, but not eliminating it. Possibly preventing its onset, but not fixing a pancreas that hasn't worked for fifteen years. I don't want Doug to hope for a cure either.

It could be much worse, I told him one time. I could have incurable cancer or MS or a spinal cord injury. I can live with diabetes. I told him it's a blessing compared to some afflictions. And I sometimes think I was lucky to get it as a child. I was forced to adjust and didn't have the power to resist at the age of nine. It made my family closer, maybe made my mom and dad better parents. They loved me every minute I was growing up.

My childhood is the last thing I think about as I drift completely under. The plaid couch my father sat on as I crawled around him with my Barbie dolls. The way my brother cocked his head to the side when he was being scolded by my mother for biting me. His hair was thick and black and he had a lisp. I remember my sister's prom dresses and running her lipstick over my own little lips when no one was watching. I think about my parents and the way they used to laugh at us. We made them laugh and we made them yell. Denise, Brian, and I are the memories of their lives, the thoughts that carry them into old age. I'm asleep before I can think to cry.

Anger

"Just sit down," I groan, curling onto my side.

But Doug isn't hearing me. He dashes around the room with the cordless phone in one hand and my coat in the other. The 911 operator has placed him on hold for what seems like several minutes. His hands tremble as he slows to a pace. When the woman returns to the line, he tells her about my sudden attack of abdominal pain. I know she's stalling him with questions.

I shoot a frustrated look at the telephone receiver. "Just tell her I'm diabetic." I know that will speed them up.

He relays the information to the operator. She says someone will be right over. I wait, minutes feeling like hours, as pain shoots through my abdomen.

"Sit down," I say. The need to calm him overwhelms me, but the agony keeps me pinned to the floor. I'm afraid to move. It must be a complication from the tubal ligation a few weeks ago. Visions of an infection spreading through my ovaries run through my head. Maybe appendicitis. My sister had her appendix removed when she was my age. Doug continues to pace the living room floor. I watch as his leather loafers move back and forth across the hardwood floor, stopping and tapping nervously in front of the window. He pushes his face close to the glass and peers into the darkness.

"Where the hell are they?" he asks.

Within minutes, sirens are wailing down our street. The last time an ambulance pulled into our driveway, my sister had died. I roll my eyes, knowing the neighbors will be peering out their darkened windows soon. A trio of men dressed in blue come through the back door. They hover over me while Doug details my complaints. Finally, one steps forward.

"Does it hurt here?" he asks, pressing firmly on my lower abdomen.

I cringe and nod. It feels like he twisted a knife in my stomach, and I widen my eyes at him. The man in blue continues to question me about the pain: where it is, sharp or dull, continuous or erratic. I can only reply by wrapping my arms around my stomach. I can't tell the man anything specific, only that it hurts.

The three men seem inexperienced. The stretcher bounces as they stumble down the back steps and load me into the ambulance. I listen as they ask Doug irrelevant questions. They wonder about what medications I'm on, ask what I ate for dinner. They're not sure which street to turn down as they make their way back toward the city. I open my eyes to see two men exchanging knowing glances.

I'm momentarily engulfed in darkness. Unsure if I'm blacking out due to low blood sugar or the pain, I ask the man on my right to test my blood sugar.

"In just a minute there, hon."

I open my eyes wide and stare into his. *Hon?*

"Test my fucking blood sugar, now," I say between clenched teeth.

He raises his eyebrows and gives me a patronizing look before patting my right arm and telling me he'll be getting to that in just another minute. I should rest and let them worry about the situation.

I am trapped in the back of this ambulance with two technicians younger than myself who seem to know nothing about diabetes. My skin is crawling and my blood sugar must be plummeting. I know if they don't give me some sugar soon, I'm going to pass out. I focus on staying conscious. Doug is in his RX7 behind the flashing ambulance, and I want to open the back doors and get into his car with him. Drive to a convenience store and get some orange juice.

"Test my blood and give me some sugar," I tell them again.

"She's not very coherent," one of them says.

I almost laugh, but tears are starting to roll down the side of my cheek, dripping onto the lumpy pillow beneath my head. Finally I feel a lancet pricking my finger and hear the beep of the glucometer.

"No, wait a second to put the blood on," the man on my right tells the technician holding the small machine.

"I know what I'm doing," he replies defensively.

"You have to wait for the second beep. I'm telling you, man."

I enter into the conversation through a cloud.

"I can't fucking believe you two," I say. "Push the button, wait till it says to enter the strip, and then wait until it says to put the blood on. Jesus Christ." My face is hot with rage.

Finally the machine beeps three times and the tech on my right stares at the screen on the small machine. He lowers his voice and speaks across me.

"Is twenty-nine low?" he asks his partner.

"Twenty-nine is comatose, asshole," I interrupt.

Low blood sugars have made me belligerent and temperamental ever since I was a kid. I might snap at a waitress, demanding orange juice immediately, or yell at my dog because I can't find a banana in the house. I feel like I can't control my anger when my blood sugar is low. But now my fate is resting in the hands of two idiots, and I may lose consciousness because I can't get my hands on a packet of sugar. I hate these men.

"Don't you have any glucose in this place?" I ask, looking around at the metal walls.

"Uh, yeah," one of them replies, lifting the latch on a box.

His voice is full of nervous tension now. He's scared of screwing up. I listen to him rummage through the contents of the box.

"A candy bar? Anything?" I ask, trying to avoid giving them the satisfaction of hearing any desperation in my voice. "Don't you keep your little snacks in here? Didn't your mom pack you a Little Debbie or anything today?"

These men think I'm difficult, but I don't care. My tone is justified.

"Got it," the man on my left says.

He squeezes pure glucose from a clear tube into my mouth. I cough, spitting the slime out and reaching up to wipe it off my lips.

"It's all we have." He hesitates, turning the tube over in his hand. "You better take it."

The ambulance screeches to a stop. The technicians jump up and push the doors open, behaving for the first time as if they actually have an emergency on their hands. I close my eyes and pray someone inside the hospital will help me. The bumpy ride through the emergency room makes the pain in my abdomen sharper. Now it's a bleeding pain, moving from one spot and spreading throughout my gut. I open my eyes and see a nurse dressed in white. Her dress blends into the walls of this room.

Relief spreads over me. My body goes limp and I surrender to the woman standing over me. I trust that she will understand my situation and help me. I'm wrong.

"Where's the pain?" she asks in an annoyed voice.

I rest my hand on my lower abdomen and tell her I'm a diabetic and need sugar. My words sound like they were being read straight from a Medic Alert bracelet.

"Down here?" she asks, placing her hand too firmly on top of mine.

"Yeah. I need to get some sugar."

"I'll order a glucose test," she replies.

"I know it's low," I groan. I'm defeated. "The men in the

ambulance already checked it. Can't you just get me some orange juice?"

I'm still talking as she turns away and pulls the curtain closed behind her. Doug walks in.

"What a bitch," I say to him. "Did you see that woman?"

He looks around the curtain into an empty hallway and shakes his head, wondering what caused the irritation in my voice.

I try to tell myself the nurse was only doing her job. Normally, I sympathize with doctors and nurses. Even though they treat diabetics every day, they must accommodate the idiosyncrasies of each of us. Diabetes is a defined illness. That's the problem. Medical personnel are trained to deal with the textbook cases, the most common problems associated with diabetes. They are taught the magic numbers for high and low blood sugars, and they learn about insulin dosages. They have studied how the body works and how it doesn't work in a diabetic patient. I trust that most of them understand the disease itself. It's the individual diabetics who aren't understood. They treat us all the same. Maybe I made no sense to the nurse a moment ago. I convince myself it was a misunderstanding.

"Did you bring my purse?" I ask Doug.

He holds it up.

"Dig around in there and find me a piece of candy."

He sits down on the edge of the chair next to my bed and rummages through the bag.

I lean forward and join him in digging around the bag. The nurse walks back in. The permanent frown on her face is transformed into a look of shock.

"What are you two doing?" she asks.

I ignore her.

"Check down at the very bottom. I think there's a peppermint somewhere down there," I tell Doug.

Through the corner of my eye, I watch as the nurse steps forward. "I told you we'd get you glucose after we run a blood test."

My eyes are fixed on a dirty, mangled piece of candy Doug is pulling from my purse. He holds it in his hand and hesitates, looking from the nurse's eyes to mine.

"I am strongly advising you not to consume that piece of candy," she says, suddenly professional.

Doug stares down at the peppermint and peels the wrapper off.

"If there is a gastrointestinal problem, consuming that might put you in jeopardy. We don't know what's wrong with you yet."

I turn my eyes to the woman. She is huge. Almost six feet tall and thick. Her hips push at the seams of the nurse's uniform and her ankles are swollen. I stare into her eyes, challenging her. The clock on the wall behind her ticks. Her words are a threat.

"Let me fill you in here," I begin. Blood is rushing to my head, and I'm suddenly filled with energy. "I have a pain in my stomach that has become unbearable. I think my appendix has probably burst, but, believe it or not, I'm not really too concerned about that right now. I had a blood sugar in that damn ambulance of twenty-nine and I haven't eaten anything for five hours. I'm sure by now my blood sugar is even lower and I'm probably only still awake because I fear that you people would let me die if I passed out. So," I continue as if I were her supervisor, "our first priority is getting my blood sugar up so I have the energy to deal with you fucking people."

Everything is silent now. My own words hang in the air around me. I can no longer hear the patients in the other rooms or phones ringing in the background. The look on the nurse's face is pure rage. Her eyes pierce through me before she turns around and storms out.

I've never spoken to a stranger so harshly, and Doug is shocked. He stares at me in disbelief but says nothing. He finishes peeling the wrapper off the piece of candy and slides it into my mouth. I try to breathe. I want out of here, but a doctor will be in to see me any minute. I know he will be as outraged as I am by what's happened.

"I'm Dr. Arnt," a man finally announces, pushing the curtain aside and walking in.

I nod and quickly size him up. His glasses are sitting crooked on his face, and his black hair is slicked back, exposing his balding head. He stares over the clipboard with threatening eyes.

"This attitude is certainly going to have to change right now," he states flatly. "It's going to be a very long night if you don't start cooperating."

Adrenaline rushes through my body, and I know the next words I choose will determine how the remaining hours in this hospital are spent. He waits for me to respond, and it seems like several minutes pass before I speak again. I rationalize that I have two options. I can either apologize and politely explain what's wrong with me, or I can explode.

"Attitude?" I ask. "Attitude? This is the first time you've even seen me. What do you know about my attitude?"

He ignores my words and gives me a look that says all his suspicions about me have just been confirmed. The nurse hadn't misinformed him. I am the uncooperative brat she described me to be.

"We can do this two ways," he begins. "Easy or hard."

"All I'm asking for is some sugar," I tell him. "That's all I've been asking for since I got here. And you people really annoy the shit out of me when my blood sugar is this low."

"Yes, I understand that," he says. "We're waiting for the blood tests to confirm your glucose level."

Something snaps in my head.

"No one has even been here to take my blood," I tell him, holding up all ten of my fingers to show him they haven't been pricked by any of the nurses here.

Shock spreads over his face and he looks to his clipboard for some explanation.

"I can't believe this," I breathe as I push myself up onto my elbow. I shove the thin white hospital blanket off my legs and painfully curl into a sitting position. I stare at Doug. "We're leaving," I state matter-of-factly, holding my abdomen. "We're gonna walk right out of this sorry excuse for an emergency room. Away from this sorry excuse for a doctor." I raise my arm in the doctor's direction.

I can tell from the look on Doug's face that he doesn't know how to respond. He looks up at the balding man holding the clipboard and then back to me struggling to make my way off the bed. He hesitates before taking my arm.

"Just trust me, honey," I tell him. "We're not staying here. I'm not going to let this man put his hands on me."

I'm overwhelmed with the strangest sensation. The feeling that if this doctor touches me I'm going to die. If he gets his hands on me he will intentionally hurt me. I need to leave.

"Let's just wait a minute," Doug says. "There could really be something wrong and we probably shouldn't leave here."

"Listen to him," the doctor interjects, nodding toward Doug.

I shoot the man a look of warning and pull my coat off the back of Doug's chair. I grab Doug's hand and pull my purse onto my shoulder. The bag slams against my back. I wrap my other arm around my stomach and walk past the doctor. He follows us out.

"Where did you park?" I ask Doug.

"This way," he says, leading me down a corridor.

I lean against Doug. My legs feel like they can't carry me down the long hall. The doctor's footsteps quicken behind us. The big nurse has joined him and they are following us, talking in hushed tones. They're going to try to keep me here. I push myself forward like I'm running for my life.

"Where are you going?" the doctor asks.

I pull on Doug's sleeve to keep him moving forward. But something in me wants to stop. I want to stop and turn around and tell the doctor that he is the most despicable human being

I've ever encountered. I want to tell him that I feel sorry for the people who come through the doors of this emergency room and are met by him. A part of me wants to scream at him, and another part of me wants to drop to the floor and let him take care of me. But the initial fear of his placing his hands on me forces me forward to the exit door.

As the car door shuts behind me, I breathe a sigh of relief. Doug drives me straight to Quik Trip and buys a carton of orange juice. I force the entire carton down my throat as he heads for another hospital. The headlights of other cars blind me. I want to laugh. I feel like a fugitive, but I know I'm going to be all right now. I clutch the carton close to my chest. I regain control over myself. Over my life.

"Turn left here," I tell Doug. We're going to Des Moines General.

"Okay." He glances over at me. "Still hurt a lot?"

I nod. The pain is starting to subside, but each time the car hits a bump I feel the jolt through my abdomen.

"I'm afraid it's from the tubal," I say. "I can't believe what just happened."

"I don't know, Andie. You were being pretty nasty to those people."

"What?" I start to shake. "*I* was nasty to *them*? Do you realize what just happened back there? They would have been responsible if I had gone unconscious."

Doug doesn't argue with me. He knows it will only make me more upset if he challenges my behavior in the hospital. He's seen my reaction to doctors and nurses when I'm angry. When I had the preliminary physical for my vitrectomy, Doug said I was rude to the nurse taking blood from my arm. The woman missed the vein the first time, and I rolled my eyes. When she dug the point into my skin the second time and missed, I told her to call someone else. I asked her if she had a technician who knew how to do it. I didn't mean to insult her, but she looked offended. When she walked out of the room, Doug told me I had been mean. I replied that he wasn't the one sitting on the white cot getting his arm jabbed.

We drive in silence to the second hospital, where they immediately run an ultrasound and tell me I have two ruptured cysts on my ovary. The doctor gives me pills for the pain and antibiotics. She tells me cysts are common, but the ones on my ovary had been very large. When they broke, they caused intense pain that spread throughout my abdomen.

On the way home, Doug maneuvers through the streets of Des Moines toward the interstate. The pain medication makes me drowsy, but I'm still angry. I pull my hair on top of my head and let my body sink into the leather seat. Doug reaches across me and pulls the seat belt around my chest. He clicks it into place before securing his own. He takes care of me, but he can't really understand what I'm feeling. He hasn't dealt with doctors as I have. He's still amazed that we walked out of the first hospital. He is not sure why I spoke to the nurse and doctor the way I did. I want to complain that people think doctors are gods. People die because they believe their doctors are all-knowing and have the final word on everything. We forget that our bodies belong to us no matter what emergency room we're being wheeled into.

The older I get, the more I understand why my mother yelled at the doctors in the hospital when Denise and I were children. She was trying to take some control in a situation where it seemed she didn't have any. She resented their authority. She learned to rely on herself, pick and choose the advice she was given about her daughters. Now I have to do the same thing. I have to listen to the doctors, but I can't depend on them for everything. I have to trust them, but I have to trust myself more.

When Doug pulls into the driveway, I don't move. The radio has stopped playing, the engine isn't humming. Just the two of us in the dark car in complete silence. I stare at the front door of the house, still angry but relieved that my condition wasn't more serious. Doug unfastens his seat belt and leans toward me. Instead of fumbling for words, he brushes my hair away from my face. He's content to sit here all night with me and stare at the house if I want to. I suppress the urge to complain about the first doctor again. He would listen, but the silence is too perfect.

Satin Slippers

I CAN FEEL MY father looking at me as I stare at myself in the mirror. I push the headband of my veil down firmly against my hair, resting my fingers for a moment on the curves of the white braid. My mother insisted on making the veil herself and wove beads and lace through the hairpiece before fitting it perfectly to my head. My fingernails are coated with clear polish, and I try unsuccessfully to steady my hands. I check my lipstick and smooth the front of my white dress. Its narrow lace sleeves lightly scratch my arms. The flowing skirt brushes the tops of my satin shoes. Ann tried to talk me into buying white heels, but I insisted on slippers. I look like a small child playing dress-up in her mother's gown. And in a way, I am. Today I'm somewhere between childhood and adulthood. Between leaving home and building a home of my own.

The antique clock on the wall ticks. 12:48. Twelve minutes. I have twelve minutes to wait. Twelve minutes to talk to my father before we walk through a room filled with people. Looking into the mirror at the reflection of the dressing room, I see a painting of a woman making bread. Other paintings in thick oak frames are bolted to the walls. Eyes burn at me from all directions. I look at my father's reflection. He is leaning against the door frame, staring at me.

"Are you nervous?" I ask.

"All the attention is going to be on you," he replies with a hint of sarcasm.

"That tux transforms you into a pretty handsome guy." I wink into the mirror.

He looks younger today, but perhaps the tuxedo just makes me think of high school proms. The black suit fits him perfectly, and the burgundy vest brings color to his January complexion. His hands are folded in front of him, and he waits patiently, like a man who has no worries, no schedule to keep. But the clock ticks. My palms are sweating. My first reaction is to wipe them on the front of my dress, but I resist the urge. This dress has transformed me for the day. I want to say something to my father. Something meaningful before I make the transition into being a wife.

I focus on myself in the mirror, trying to find the words. I want to tell him that Doug will take care of me. I want to thank my dad for teaching me about integrity and goodness. I want to tell him he has done his job well, more than fulfilled the obligations of a father. But words like these would sound too final. I listen to the people file in below me. Bits and pieces of conversations float up the stairs.

"I wonder how many people won't make it because of the weather," I say. It's the coldest day of the year in Iowa. Even though the sun is shining, the extreme temperatures are causing the batteries in cars to go dead. Ten inches of blowing snow yesterday kept my aunts and uncles from Minneapolis home. "I guess this was the risk of a January wedding," I say.

When he nods I notice a sadness in his eyes. He's growing old before me, almost shriveling in his formal attire. His eyes seem to belong to a man who thinks the world is out of reach but has accepted it. In a few minutes he will watch me vow to depend on and cherish another man for the rest of my life. But there has to be some comfort in that. I want him to find some comfort in knowing that I'll never be alone. He just looks sad now. He's dressed in the black suit to give me to another man.

The progression of life pushes me forward, away from my father.

I wonder if my sister is watching me today. She would like my dress. I've been thinking a lot about Denise the last few months, wondering if she ever regretted not getting married. Wondering if she would be surprised to know that I'm doing it. She would have liked Doug, and if she were still alive, she would be the one standing next to me today. I like believing she's with me anyway, somehow hovering above it all and smiling. I look at my father, spot a tear in the corner of his eye.

I've never seen him cry. Not real tears that fell down his cheeks. During my sister's funeral, he stared straight ahead and chewed on his top lip. Sometimes his eyes would gloss over, but he blinked the tears away or turned his head. The same Unitarian minister who performed Denise's funeral service is performing my wedding ceremony today. When Doug and I wrote our ceremony, we included some of the readings from my sister's funeral. It is my way of bringing Denise into my future. Carrying her memory with me as I go on with my life.

"Did Denise ever talk to you about getting married?" I ask.

"Not that I remember." He clears his throat and looks up at the ceiling, thinking. "There was that one man when she was in graduate school. His name was Steve, I think. I thought they might get married, but she never said anything about it. I guess she just didn't meet the right person."

I search my memory for a Steve. I don't remember my sister ever talking about marriage.

"The last time we saw all these people together in one place was at her funeral, you know?" I say.

He nods.

Denise's funeral was harder on my father than on anyone. He had turned and walked away from the crowd as the minister spoke by her grave. One of my mother's friends was handing out roses to set on Denise's casket. Everyone except my father placed the flowers on the silver box. My dad held his close to his chest and walked down the hill to the road. Leaning against the back of the limousine, he stared at the red flower and waited for us to say our good-byes.

I lift my bouquet of roses from the vanity and bring them close to my face. White and red roses with baby's breath and ivy woven through them. White beads hang from the base of the bouquet, blending into my dress. I turn the arrangement in my hands and study it from all angles. I will toss it to Ann at the reception later. I'll stand with my back to the line of my single friends and throw it to the right side where she'll be standing. The band will be playing loudly, and no one will know we've planned it.

My mother said she hopes we don't do anything crazy today. No kidnapping the bride, no smashing cake into each other's faces. No rice. Even rigging the bouquet toss with Ann would make her shake her head in disgust. I won't tell her. Plans for this wedding have consumed my mother for months. Everything has been perfectly organized. The limousine is waiting outside, bows are tied to the backs of chairs downstairs. My mother has remembered every detail. It's like she's waited for these next thirty minutes her whole life. The party after the ceremony will be a relief.

The reception hall seems a world away. I would rather be there, away from the formality and nervous tension of the formal ceremony. My relatives decorated the huge room last night with balloons and streamers. They hung pictures of Doug and me as children on the walls. The manager of the hall told us we couldn't use Scotch tape, so my mother bought packages of a yellow gumlike substance. It didn't work. The decorations kept sliding down the walls. My mother stared at the mess around her and scrambled up the nearest chair to negotiate the streamers. Sweat ran down her neck as she ran around the hall. She acted like a kid again, barking orders at her brothers and sisters. I was calm last night, comforted by the obvious fact that she was worrying enough for the both of us. Now my heart beats hard against the bouquet pulled close to my chest.

"I bet the pictures the photographer took are going to turn out great," I say, changing the subject.

"It's a beautiful place here," he replies. My father never says anything that isn't genuine.

After searching for weeks, Doug and I chose to be married in this museum. Neither of us belongs to a church. This mansion was built in 1877 by General William Sherman's brother. The famous general from the Civil War visited for parties and social gatherings with dignitaries. Music from the baby grand piano drifts up the staircase.

I wonder if my father is remembering his own wedding. He and my mom were married in the Little Brown Church in northern Iowa. They eloped because my father's family didn't approve of their marriage. But they're still together after all this time. I think they love each other, but they never kiss anymore. I fear that about marriage. I fear routine and monotony, even though it seems unthinkable now. I want to ask my father what he was thinking about on the day he married my mom. Everything was so different back then—my parents drove 300 miles to a bowling tournament for their honeymoon. Doug and I are flying to Cancún. I look like my mother in her wedding pictures. Her veil pulled her dark hair away from her rounded face too. Everyone says I look like my mother now.

"How have your eyes been lately?" my father asks, glancing up at the clock.

I don't want to talk about my eyes, but I expect this question from him at least once a week.

I always tell him they're doing better.

"When is your next appointment in Iowa City?" he asks.

"Two weeks. Two weeks from Monday."

"I can drive you, you know. We'll stop and have lunch on the way."

I nod, knowing Doug will be taking me from now on. He has already requested the day off work. My father took me to all the appointments before I met Doug.

"The blood from the vitrectomy looks like it's almost all settled out," he comments.

"There's still a little around the sides," I say, touching the corner of my eye. "They told me in some people it will never completely clear. It's been months, and that eye still gets irritated easily."

I run my pinkie under the eye, careful not to smear the mascara. I am still embarrassed about the blood circling my iris, and I tilted my head to the side in the pictures the photographers took this morning. I want to remember the day of my wedding, not the surgery.

"No one else notices, though," he reassures me.

"I guess." I pause. "So are you okay with all this?"

"All what?" he asks.

"Me getting married to Doug."

"Of course." He sounds surprised I've asked. "I always knew you would find the right one eventually."

"I just want you to know that he's a really great guy. He's the kind of guy who will be there whenever I need him because he wants to be, not just because he has to be. I can't really explain it, I just know it. My gut tells me he's genuine."

"I know," he replies.

"I don't want you to think that I don't need you or anything now." The words don't come easily, and I wipe a tear from the corner of my right eye.

"I know, sweetie." He walks over to me and straightens the back of my veil. He leans against me and whispers in my ear. "We better get down there, Andie."

I take one last look in the mirror and turn around. As I take my father's arm, we turn and head down the stairs.

My friend Holly walks ahead of us, pausing at the end of the aisle and looking straight up as the photographers told her to.

I grab my father's arm more tightly and straighten out the bottom of my dress.

"We have to pause at the back here before we walk up, Dad. Virginia said to do that so she can get our picture."

"Okay," he whispers.

When Holly gets to the minister, she turns to face the back of the room. Ann steps forward and smiles as she walks slowly. Her parents are sitting in the last row, and her mom smiles beneath the tears when she sees Ann.

As I step to the left of my father, I scan the crowd of family and friends. They smile back at me and stand up in unison. Tears well in my eyes as I study their faces. Holly told me that the happiest moment of her wedding was when she stood at the end of the aisle. She started to cry when everyone stood up. She said she felt that everyone loved her so much. It was like having God in the room.

I face forward and look straight up the long aisle at Doug. He smiles when he sees my father and me, and I walk more quickly, wanting to get to him as fast as I can. Images of my past fill my head. The cakes my mother made me on my birthdays, playing hide-and-seek with my brother, the way my father looked at me when I graduated from college. I add the image of myself walking down the aisle to my collection of memories, and the tension in my back diminishes.

My father gives Doug my arm. Doug extends his right arm to shake hands with my father, and I wonder if the minister told him before the ceremony to do this. We didn't have a rehearsal last night, and we are all unsure about what we are supposed to be doing up here. Holly is gazing at the minister's hands. She's probably locked her knees. Ann's head is tilted affectionately as she watches us. Out of the corner of my eye, I spot my mother in the front row. She's smiling and wiping her eyes. My brother has his arm around her shoulders. My father shakes Doug's hand and steps back to take his seat next to my mother.

A child giggles in the background and a mother whispers for

him to be quiet. When I take Doug's hand the roomful of people disappear. I feel the overwhelming joy I've been waiting for. Waiting my whole life for. For one moment I forget about the eye surgeries, forget my fear of blindness. Everything is okay. Doug looks down at my white gown and squeezes my hand. The minister opens the ceremony and the familiar words ring in my ears. I speak the words loudly, making promises to both Doug and myself about our future. When we wrote the ceremony, he had insisted on adding a promise to my vows. He wanted me to promise that I would allow him to love me. He said that's more important to him than anything. So I run my fingers over his wedding band and say that I will.

Forming Lines with the Snow

LAST NIGHT's blizzard has left the ground blanketed in snow. I am met with only rolling white hills. The landmarks that show me the way to her grave in warmer months are covered. Everything looks the same, and there are no footprints but my own as I follow a narrow row of trees up the hill. I know she's buried near the seventh tree, but I'm unsure of exactly where I am. I kneel to brush flakes off unfamiliar grave markers and move more quickly up the incline on my hands and knees in search of my sister. My heart pounds beneath the layers of winter clothing. Each cold gray rock I uncover disappoints me with a name I don't know. My fingers go numb beneath my thin gloves. Sometimes I imagine that her death has been a dream. I come here to remind myself that she's never coming back.

Finally, my hand wipes away the heavy flakes covering my sister's name. DENISE IRENE DOMINICK. 1959 to 1993. I breathe the cold, dry air deep into my lungs and lower myself onto the undisturbed snow where the casket was buried. I remove my glove and trace the engraving of her name with my finger. The limestone marker still looks brand new. Wind blows dusty snow against my face. I pull the hood of my coat tightly around my ears and turn my eyes up to the rest of the cemetery.

I'm surrounded by dead bodies. I am the only breathing creature as far as I can see. A silence of deserted land surrounds me. People don't visit the cemetery in February. Christmas has passed and the groundskeepers have removed the plastic ever-greens and wreaths placed on the graves by mothers. My mother decorates this spot every December. She puts a tiny tree with plastic bulbs in the pop-up vase, but she comes back after the holidays and takes it home again. She wraps it in a plastic bag and places it on an old wooden shelf in their basement.

I push my hand down into the snow and touch the hard ground beneath me, wondering how they break the earth when someone dies in February. The obituary section of the news-paper has been full the last few weeks. Car accidents and heart attacks. A man on a farm outside Des Moines murdered his two children and wife before shooting himself. A young black woman was kidnapped and found dead several days later. A semitrailer truck slid across the median strip on the interstate and hit an oncoming Honda. A mother and both her daughters were killed. The ground must be harder to penetrate for caskets in the winter. Denise died in July after heavy rains.

The day of her funeral seems an eternity ago, and covered in snow this place is not familiar. I have only seen it green and full of life. I chose her plot next to these small trees that humid sum-mer day, but now they have no leaves. They have gone dormant for the winter. Heavy icicles cling to their branches as they wait for spring to arrive. The trees stand alone with no shelter from the bitter cold and surrender to the wind.

"Well, here we are." I pause to recognize the sound of my own voice breaking the silence. "It seems like there's so much I should tell you. I've been doing a lot lately. Got married, bought a house, got a dog. I'll be finishing my Master's in a few more months, and then I don't know. You would like Doug though."

The wind blows harder against my face, and I lower my head into my hands.

"The house is really big, but you wouldn't believe it if you saw it. It's pink. Not just painted pink but pink siding and a pink garage and pink carpet inside. You know how I hate pink, so I suppose we'll be doing a lot of work the next few months."

It was hard moving out of the house I'd lived in with Denise. As I packed the boxes, I thought about all I had experienced in those rooms. I felt like I was abandoning the memories of my sister. I cleaned out the closets and the shed, coming across things of hers I hadn't seen in years. Her leather gloves were pushed to the back of the hall closet behind the vacuum cleaner. Pages from her Master's thesis turned up in my file cabinet. The gloves were ragged and the pages were yellowing, and I finally threw them into the black trash bag with my other garbage. It felt okay to let everything go.

I needed to start fresh with Doug. The house was my way of holding on to my life before I met him. My life with my sister and then the years without her. Sometimes I'm glad Doug never knew her. He doesn't even realize how much he forces me to live in the present. I think about my sister every day, but she doesn't linger in my head the way she used to. I'm not the same person now. I still hesitate for a moment when people ask me how many siblings I have, but I don't become lost in thought as I did the first year after she was gone. It's not really any easier, it's just different now. Being with Doug makes me realize how much time has passed, how far I've come.

"Sometimes it feels like I still don't really fit anywhere though. It's like I'm waiting for something that other people aren't waiting for. Waiting for something to go wrong. To go blind or die or for my kidneys to fail. I can't make sense of it. I had another vessel break in my eye last week. All these surgeries and you would think they could get it right by now. I was just helping Doug move a couch in the living room when it happened." The cold air stings my lungs when I inhale. "Other days I have moments when everything is clear. I know for an instant that it's all going to be okay. Everything will work out. Then that feeling passes and I can't recapture it."

I pull my hand away from my face and place it on the stone. "There are moments when I miss you so much. I missed you at the wedding when I looked back at the front row. Mom and Dad were both crying. I kept thinking you had to be back there somewhere watching me. I didn't think you'd miss it." I shake my head and stare into the snow.

I feel strange now, sitting on the cold ground talking to myself. I straighten up for a better view of the cemetery. A green sedan is parked next to the pond. A father and daughter are climbing a steep hill that levels off near their car. As her father drags the sled behind him, the small child skips ahead in anticipation. When they reach the top, he pulls her stocking cap down over her ears and helps her onto the sled. Then he watches from the top as she wraps her mittens around the plastic handles and descends. Her laughter breaks the silence, brings life to this place. The wind rushes through her hair, and she's oblivious to the occasional bump of a grave marker on her way down. She doesn't realize that she's gliding over dead bodies.

My stomach rumbles deep beneath my down parka, and I lick my cracking lips.

"I think Mom was crying because of you. Every time she cries now, I think it's because of you. A sad movie comes on and she starts to weep, and I think to myself that it's just an excuse to shed some tears." I shake my head. "I mean she never cried like this when we were growing up. Now she cries at the drop of a hat."

I look back toward the child. With her red coat hanging below her knees, she stands at the edge of the pond and waits for her father to reach the bottom of the hill. The tall man carries a bread bag with dry slices to feed the birds in one hand and the girl's scarf in the other. The kid lost it on the way down the hill. Dragging his boots through the deep snow, he moves in slow motion. He seems tired, and his muscles are probably sore. The child looks back at her father and bends down to dip her mitten into the pond. A high-pitched squeal escapes her lips as the icy water penetrates the thick red material. Her grandmother probably made them for her.

I scan the rest of the cemetery. White. There are no other cars approaching, no movement across the empty terrain. I settle back into the snow. The heat from my legs melts the snowflakes on my jeans, and the damp denim sticks to my thighs, making me part of the ground. Everything is still. Even though the days are getting a little longer, I know it will be dark soon. I can feel the night coming.

"I'm afraid to go blind," I say. "I'm more afraid of that than anything. And being married to Doug makes it worse somehow. I don't want him to have to take care of me. I don't think I can live with being a liability. I'm scared."

I pause as if I'm expecting an answer, but I know what my sister would say. She would tell me to stop worrying about the future. It seems as if I heard her voice just days ago. And it's my voice too. I didn't realize that until a few months after she died and I called my house, letting the phone ring until the answering machine picked up so I could get my messages. I heard my voice on the line and realized it sounded like Denise's. To the point and raspy. I can hear her in myself.

"Even though he's with me, sometimes I'm so alone. But maybe it's better that way. I can't take anyone with me through the bad times anyway. Not really. I know Doug will be there, but it's still my life that I must play out. He's there, but I'm still trapped inside myself."

The little girl's laughter echoes across the open space, and I turn my head and watch her father pulling her through the snow on the sled. She's holding on with both hands and the bag of bread has been left next to the water. Two geese move forward to investigate its contents. The father spots the birds and drops the rope on the sled, moving quickly toward the plastic bag and snatching it up. The girl rolls off the sled and runs to her father, holding out her hands. He pulls a slice from the bag and hands it to her before taking out one for himself. Then he tears the piece of bread into smaller pieces and throws them into the water toward the birds. The girl drops her mittens on the ground and imitates him, laughing as the birds swim quickly toward the food. They dunk their heads beneath the surface of the icy water.

Then she reaches out her hand to take the bag from her father. He releases it and her small fingers dig into the plastic. Walking closer to the water, she glances at her dad before turning the bag upside down and dropping all the bread into the icy water at once. More birds flock to the floating slices, greedily sinking their beaks into them and tearing them apart. The sudden activity of the creatures startles the small child to tears. She turns to her father, who kneels and pulls her close to his chest.

I fed the birds here as a child. My mother brought me to the pond during my kindergarten year in school. My brother was in third grade and had to stay in school until 3:30. I got out at noon. Sometimes my mom would pick me up with a picnic lunch all packed and we would spread a blanket out on the grass and eat peanut butter sandwiches. I saved my crusts to give to the birds. Then my mother would pull out a book and turn over on her stomach. Facing the water, she could read the latest mystery novel and still keep an eye on me. I pulled turtles and fish out of the water, but she never let me take them home. When I asked her why, she just told me they belonged there. They wouldn't be happy anywhere else. She said their mothers would miss them.

I look up at the sky.

"They're really getting older, you know? I never thought I would notice them aging. I can hear Dad's knees crack as he walks down the basement stairs. Sometimes he repeats the same story to me two or three times, and I know he isn't sleeping at night. He takes medicine for his blood pressure now." A snowflake clings to my eyelashes. "Mom retired last year too. Her hair turned gray after your funeral and now it's white. She's survived so much."

Staring at the snow-covered ground around me, I remember how my parents had insisted on buying their own cemetery plots next to Denise's. They will be buried next to their daughter.

I pull my hood more tightly around my face, trying to shelter my forehead from the wind. A car door slams in the distance. The child and her father are leaving. She probably grew bored after running out of bread. The rumble of the engine fades as the car moves slowly toward the black iron gates. Wrapping my arms around my chest, I rock forward onto my knees. My legs are restless and I need to walk.

Leaving solitary footprints in the snow behind me, I head east with the wind to my back. I walk for several minutes before stopping to stare at a mound of black dirt protruding from the ground. It is half-covered with flakes, but the color of the dark earth dominates. Someone has just been buried, and the earth hasn't fully accepted the casket yet, refusing to settle down. The groundskeepers will have to wait until spring to plant grass and place a headstone there. I shake my head in disgust, despising the look of a fresh grave. Nothing is complete for the dead or the living as they wait for the mound of dirt to sink back down and level out. I turn back in the direction of my car.

I approach the road in front of Denise's grave and hesitate. My toes are numb in my canvas tennis shoes, and the shelter of my car looks inviting, but I turn back up the hill. Dusty snow is being blown back over the headstones I cleaned off earlier. The cemetery is returning to its undisturbed state. The footprints I left are fading, but I follow what's left of my presence up the hill and find her name immediately. I sit down again and search for words.

"Well, it's pretty cold out here. I should probably go home to my husband now." I feel a smile appear on my lips. "Doesn't that sound strange? After we got married, I kept saying the word *wife* over and over. It feels strange to be someone's wife."

Doug is probably worried about me. I told him I was running a few errands and would be home by early afternoon. A fire is burning in the fireplace, and he's probably listening to talk radio and doing the Saturday cleaning without me. I know he's glancing at his watch every few minutes and wondering what's taking me so long.

"I wish you could meet him," I sigh. "He's really unbelievable. He's the one you would have picked for me if you were here. Sometimes it's tough though. Being married is harder than being single ever was. He always says to me, 'We're on the same team.' I understand that, and I'm trying to learn how to be a team player. Sometimes it doesn't seem anyone can really be on my team." I pause. "Except for you, I guess."

I reach out and form lines with the snow on her stone. Thin rows of white flakes.

"I guess I won't be buried here, next to you now, huh? I don't know. I suppose Doug and I will buy plots together or something. It doesn't really matter, does it? Where I'm buried, I mean." I pause. "Dee Dee, I have to get home now." I stand up and turn my back to her grave.

Snow is coming down harder, and the flakes stick to the windows of my car as I turn up the heat. I lean my head against the back of the seat and look in the direction of her grave. The white snow makes the spots in my eyes more prominent, but a sense of peace surrounds me. Something blowing across the pavement catches my eye. The wind carries a plastic bread bag over the graves.